Finding Happiness after Covid-19

Towards a new and better normal

Dr Pam and Peter Keevil

Dedication

To all those people whose transformative practices we have
used over the years

Table of Contents

Disclaimer

The views in this book are based on our personal experiences
only and do not claim to represent all the research and
teaching that is available at the moment

Foreword

When the Covid-19 pandemic emerged in the early months of 2020, no one could have foreseen how quickly our lives would change. Things that rightly or wrongly we had taken for granted such as travel, popping out to the pub, booking tickets for the theatre, or simply sitting in a café watching the world go by disappeared. It was right to feel fearful, sad, angry, annoyed, resentful or whatever else you personally felt. It was right, too, to question what was being done as we were all in uncharted territory and no one knew when the end would come. And when it did, would we be able to go back to our former lifestyle? Could we, as a society or as an individual, afford to? More importantly, would we want to? If not, what was this new and better normal that we would prefer to create and move onto?

The feeling of unreality as events were cancelled and life put on hold and we faced an uncertain future created pain, fear and disbelief. Some people would describe this as alienation, a disconnect from what is happening around them.

The purpose of this book is to help people find a way to make the changes we'll all need to make, as we emerge from the first wave of Covid-19; and to seek to create a new and better normal way of life. We also wanted to write this book to provide information, ideas and resources to organisations and communities to develop their resilience and well being for a post Covid-19 world.

The first thing is to decide what we really want from this gift of life.

We are human *beings*, not human *doings,* and human *beings* rather than human *buyings*

Introduction

Until Covid-19 hit us and radically changed our lives, we might have thought that most people in our society would have enjoyed more happiness than any previous generations. We acknowledge that there are still sections of our society and our world who struggle to survive. However, for many of us, we've grown accustomed to the benefits of Western lifestyle that until a generation ago was unimaginable. For example:

- routinely taking foreign holidays anywhere we wanted
- buying a new or more up to date car
- going out to gastro pubs and restaurants
- going to festivals, to the theatre, cinema
- going shopping and "do the sales"
- responding via our credit cards to the welter of adverts that have bombarded us

Of course, we don't have data on how happy our ancestors were, but we do have recent data on happiness (pre Covid-19) in most countries. The best source of data on happiness country by country comes from the Gallup World Poll. The data shows that the happiest countries are in Scandinavia. In 2019, the UK was ranked 15th for happiness in the world, according to the annual World Happiness Report (www.worldhappinessreport/ed/2019).

There's also data now for specific countries showing the trends over time. In the US, people are no happier now than they were in the 1950s, despite huge improvements in living standards there (Layard, 2020). Research by Jean Twenge of San Diego State University shows that the years since 2010 have not been good ones for happiness and well-being among Americans. Even as the United States economy improved after the end of the Great Recession in 2009, happiness among adults did not rebound to the higher levels of the 1990s, continuing a slow decline ongoing since at least 2000 in the General Social Survey (Twenge et al., 2016). Happiness and life satisfaction among United States adolescents, which increased between 1991 and 2011, suddenly declined after 2012. Thus, by 2016-17, both adults and adolescents were reporting significantly less happiness than they had in the 2000s.

Globally, the data (Layard 2020) shows us that happiness has fallen in nearly as many countries as those where it has risen. He goes onto say that:

> *The extra happiness provided by extra income is greatest when you are poor, and declines steadily as you get richer*

Now that we find ourselves in a post Covid-19 world, with its economic upheavals, the abolition of our normal expectations of what we can and cannot do, coupled with the anxiety and stress that go with all of this, what chances are there of societies and individuals retaining and developing their happiness? This book provides a single source where you can find some of the greatest insights developed over decades (and in some cases, centuries) about how to be happy.

As if these challenges were not enough, there's another important angle on all this which we also want to explore: and this is the effect of our pre Covid-19 lifestyles on nature and the planet - resulting in the now well documented climate emergency. Here, the data shows us that our recent lifestyles have been threatening the health of the planet's ecosystems — we're threatening our own survival.

According to data from the Mauna Loa Observatory in Hawaii, the concentration of Co_2 in the atmosphere is over 415 parts per million (ppm), far higher than at any point in the last 800,000 years, since before the evolution of mankind.

Climate change is threatening our earth and the life it sustains. With that and the constantly growing human population, we can't afford to keep turning a blind eye to biodiversity loss. How can we possibly be happy if we've destroyed the planet, and have no food to sustain us?

In the past, happiness has often been defined in the following way:

A sense that one's life is good, meaningful, and worthwhile
(Sonya Lyubomirsky 2007)

More recently, the Action for Happiness movement (www.actionforhappiness.org), founded by Richard Layard and sponsored by the Dalai Lama has moved the happiness agenda on to include our way of life:

We want to see a fundamentally different way of life - where people care less about what they can get just for themselves and more about the happiness of others

In the light of Covid-19 and with more pandemics a distinct possibility, we believe it's time to extend the scope of happiness to include 3 key aspects:

- understanding of and compassion for ourselves as individuals
- understanding of and compassion for others
- understanding of and compassion for nature and the planet we live on

For this reason, an essential part of happiness is to seek to understand (as much as we can) these three parts of our world, to identify areas we can change and to take action.

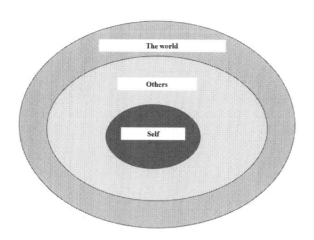

In reading this book, there are three broad approaches you might want to consider, depending on your personality and your intentions:

- the first approach is simply to read all of it, or just those parts of it that interest you most; and then, afterwards, consider what, if any, changes you would most like to take. At this stage, you might want to return to some of the earlier chapters which describe tools to help us make changes to our lives

- the second approach is to read the book in full, pausing at the various points to think about and action plan the changes you would most like in your life; and start taking actions almost from day 1

- the third approach is for organisations such as local Action for Happiness groups or branches of the Transition Movement to use it as the basis for workshops, exploring specific chapters or tools, one at a time. In the *Epilogue*, we provide details of a linked Facebook page, where people can, if they like, share, explore and discuss their thoughts about any of the issues covered in this book.

The choice is yours. We've written the book in a way that lends itself to all of these approaches.

The implications for us all in dealing with pandemics such as Covid-19 are enormous; and to an extent overwhelming. Can we ever return to the old normal – we suspect not. We will all have to adjust how we think, feel and behave in the new climate.

Fortunately, there are lots of sources of inspiration, tools and techniques which have been developed in the last fifty years or so which can help us to do exactly this. And that's why we have written this book, which represents a distillation of the *best bits* of personal development we have been privileged to access and learn about, plus lots of practical tools and techniques we can all choose to use or not, to help us adapt and create a new and better normal. These practical tools are best thought of as the contents of a Happiness Toolkit, as shown below:

Happiness Toolkit

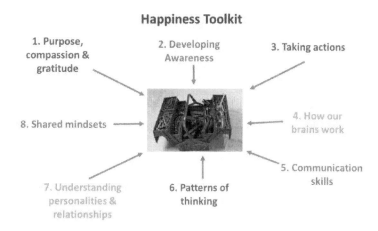

1. Purpose, compassion & gratitude

2. Developing Awareness

3. Taking actions

8. Shared mindsets

4. How our brains work

7. Understanding personalities & relationships

6. Patterns of thinking

5. Communication skills

The book is structured so that there is a specific chapter on each of these tools.

But first, we start off with having a look at the whole topic of happiness, which has been well researched now for a few years and which tells us some interesting things about how happy we actually were, even pre Covid-19.

Chapter one: What is happiness?

As we wrote in the last chapter, we believe there's a need to reconsider what happiness means to us, as individuals and in relation to other people and the world and why it's important. Richard Layard's research (Layard, 2005 and 2020) shows that there are real benefits to being happy. Happy people:

- have closer friends and are better connected with other people
- create more happiness in others
- are healthier
- bounce back better from adversity
- are more trusting, showing more compassion to themselves, others and the world

But the term *happiness* no doubt means different things to different people. For some, it's probably about those peak moments in life, such as their wedding day, the birth of a child or a special event. We recognise that some people would say it's unrealistic to imagine anyone can be happy for all, or most of their life, or maybe not for much of their life given the challenges and struggles we experience. We also recognise that many would say something like happiness is the end result of success in life... success in either getting enough money, the right job, a good place to live, the right partner and family life, i.e. it's a destination to work towards.

In this book, we interpret happiness as a deep-rooted sense of wellbeing, a set of powerful resources we can draw on to help us overcome life's challenges; a deep sense of being and feeling okay with yourself, others and the world. In our culture, the advertisements that continually bombard us tempt us with what we might call *external wealth* i.e. a bigger and better job; a bigger and better house; and a bigger and better car. These things can be important, but we would suggest that in addition to this *external wealth,* there is another and possibly more important kind of wealth, i.e. **internal wealth.** Our internal wealth is the experience that our life is worth living, in a rewarding, engaging and meaningful way.

The essential components of internal wealth include:

- a well rooted sense of purpose in our lives; knowing our core values; and a natural instinct to use these to give a sense of direction
- an instinct for compassion – for ourselves, for others and for the world
- a sense of gratitude
- physical and mental health
- material wealth to satisfy our most basic needs

It's this kind of internal wealth that actually matters more, in helping us to achieve happiness. When we know that we have these kinds of resources, held internally, we truly know we are rich! This will be explored more fully in a later chapter.

Finally, we'll suggest that happiness is not an end destination, i.e. a consequence of working hard and being successful, but instead is the *process* we follow throughout our lives, the sequence of millions and millions of tiny actions we take each day to live our lives, and the manner and spirit we choose for each of these tiny steps.

How many people have you met in your lifetime who clearly and explicitly say they want to be unhappy? And yet, how many people do you know who can genuinely say they are really happy? And what is happiness? The first section of the book explores what this means.

The good news is that in the last twenty years or so there's been a lot of research into what happiness is, and how we can choose to respond to the world and what happens to us in a way which is likely to increase our overall level of happiness.

So, what do you think would make you happier? If we look at the bombardment of adverts we see and hear every day on the media, we might be forgiven for thinking it's:

- that dream holiday
- the festive Christmas season
- that new car
- a new kitchen
- anything that advertisers or influencers describe as a *must have*

Or might it be something deeper such as:

- losing weight
- finding a new partner
- having a child

- more money
- more time
- your child excelling at school

Nice though all such things would be, the scientific research tells us that such things can make a small difference – and sometimes quite a short-lived difference.

One researcher, Sonya Lyubomirsky, who was a professor of psychology at the University of California and is the author of *The How of Happiness* (2007) conducted research on what kinds of things tend to make us, long term, happier. What she discovered was that about fifty percent of our happiness is determined by our genetic inheritance, therefore leaving the remaining fifty percent down to our own actions, responses to life events, thoughts and feelings. A summary of her findings is found in the following graph:

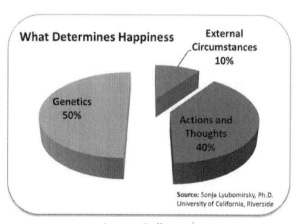

Jeremy Rolleston[i]

The research shows that a significant chunk (fifty percent) of our happiness is determined by our genetic inheritance, i.e. the way our bodies create and move around certain hormones such as serotonin. As a result, it makes sense to work on the forty percent that is in our control; our actions and thoughts.

Possibly, the most surprising part of this research is that only a tiny fraction (ten percent) of our happiness is determined by what Sonya Lyubomirsky calls *external circumstances* i.e. those things we often most strive for; the new job, new partner, new car or dream holiday. There is a lot of science which backs this up. Sonya Lyubomirsky's work includes one study in America which showed that the richest people – those earning millions of dollars, report levels of happiness only slightly higher than the office staff and blue-collar staff they employ. Although married people are generally happier than single people, the effect of marriage on personal happiness is often quite small. For example:

> *Of married adults 40% call themselves very happy, while only 23% of never-marrieds do. This is true of every ethnic group studied, and it is true across the seventeen nations that psychologists have surveyed*
>
> (Seligman, 2002)

Richard Layard goes on in *Happiness* to explain the paradox that when individual people become richer compared with other people, they become happier. But when whole societies have become richer, they have not become happier. As the above diagram shows, it appears that about forty percent of the differences in our happiness levels are still left unexplained. What, then, are the factors that make up this forty percent? The term that Sonya Lyubomirsky uses to describe these factors is our daily intentional activities, which in the above pie chart are better described as our thoughts and feelings.

This is great news, since in theory at least, we, and only we, have control over our thoughts and feelings. The kinds of things that make up this critical forty percent are:

- having a sense of purpose in your life
- having a deep-rooted sense of compassion for yourself, for others and for the world
- expressing gratitude for all we have
- offering a helping hand to a neighbour or a friend
- living in the moment
- physical exercise and getting out into nature
- having lifelong goals and working towards them
- bouncing back from a setback

By now, you may be wondering how you compare with others in the scale of happiness. Fortunately, you're not the first person to ask this question. The following questionnaire (the Oxford Happiness Questionnaire which was designed by psychologists Michael Argyle and Peter Hills at Oxford University) has been included to give us some insights:

The Oxford Happiness Questionnaire

Below are a number of statements about happiness.

Please indicate how much you agree or disagree with each by entering a number in the blank after each statement, according to the following scale:

1 = strongly disagree 2 = moderately disagree 3 = slightly disagree 4 = slightly agree 5 = moderately agree 6 = strongly agree

Please read the statements carefully. Some of the questions are phrased positively and others negatively.
Don't take too long over individual questions; there are no "right" or "wrong" answers (and no trick questions)
The first answer that comes into your head is probably the right one for you
If you find some of the questions difficult, give the answer that is true for you in general or for most of the time.

1. I don't feel particularly pleased with the way I am. (R)
2. I am intensely interested in other people.
3. I feel that life is very rewarding.
4. I have very warm feelings towards almost everyone.
5. I rarely wake up feeling rested. (R)
6. I am not particularly optimistic about the future. (R)
7. I find most things amusing.
8. I am always committed and involved.
9. Life is good.

10. I do not think that the world is a good place. (R)

11. I laugh a lot.

12. I am well satisfied about everything in my life.

13. I don't think I look attractive. (R)

14. There is a gap between what I would like to do and what I have done. (R)

15. I am very happy.

16. I find beauty in some things.

17. I always have a cheerful effect on others.

18. I can fit in (find time for) everything I want to.

19. I feel that I am not especially in control of my life. (R)

20. I feel able to take anything on.

21. I feel fully mentally alert.

22. I often experience joy and elation.

23. I don't find it easy to make decisions. (R)

24. I don't have a particular sense of meaning and purpose in my life. (R)

25. I feel I have a great deal of energy.

26. I usually have a good influence on events.

27. I don't have fun with other people. (R)

28. I don't feel particularly healthy. (R)

29. I don't have particularly happy memories of the past. (R)

Calculate your score

Step 1

Items marked (R) should be scored in reverse. For example, if you gave yourself a "1," cross it out and change it to a

"6." Change "2" to a "5" Change "3" to a "4" Change "4" to a "3" Change "5" to a "2" Change "6" to a "1"

Step 2

*Use the changed scores for those 12 items and now add the numbers for **all** 29 questions.*

Step 3

Divide your grand total by 29. So your happiness score is the total (from step 2) divided by 29.

Interpreting your score

The lowest possible score is 1; and the highest score is 6. The average score is 4.3
You can of course take this questionnaire as many times as you like, so you might simply want to take a note of the date and the score; and after a while, especially if you are actively seeking to enhance aspects of your happiness, retake the questionnaire and compare the results.

When we analyse the 29 items in this questionnaire, we see that most of them fall clearly into one of the following 3 categories:

- sense of purpose (or lack of it)
- compassion (or lack of it)
- gratitude (or lack of it)

Based on our own experience of life, we believe that these 3 factors form the cornerstone of true happiness. We call this model the *Happiness Triangle*:

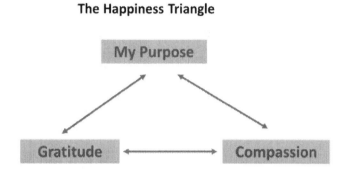

The Happiness Triangle

The 3 factors in the Happiness Triangle interact with each other in the sense that the more aware we become of the purpose in our life, the more we'll achieve; the more we achieve, the more pride we'll have; the more pride we have, the more gratitude we'll have; and the more gratitude we have, the more compassionate we'll be to self, others and the world.

We'll now go onto explore each of these 3 factors of these in turn.

Purpose: What gets us out of bed in the morning?

One international study (Garcia, 2019) found that people who have a sense of purpose in life are at lower risk of death and heart disease. Why? Researchers found that those who feel purpose often have healthier lifestyles. They are more motivated and resilient, which protects them from stress and burnout. In Japan, millions of people have *ikigai (pronounced **Ick-ee-guy)*** which is an individual's life purpose and provides a reason to jump out of bed each morning. What's your reason for getting up in the morning? Equally, studies show that losing (or not having) one's purpose can have a detrimental effect. Your *ikigai* is at the intersection of what you are good at and what you love doing.

He writes:

> ***Just as humans have lusted after objects and money since the dawn of time, other humans have felt dissatisfaction at the relentless pursuit of money and fame and have instead focused on something bigger than their own material wealth. This has over the years been described using many different words and practices, but always hearkening back to the central core of meaningfulness in life***
>
> (Garcia, 2019)

Ikigai is the convergence of at least 3 factors:

- what we're most passionate about in life
- what the world most needs
- what we're best at

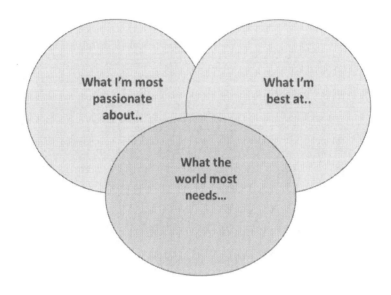

Here's an exercise you can do, which is a simplified version of Garcia's model.

Stage 1	Write down answers to the questions above and write them into the spaces in each of the circles
Stage 2	Draw a square in the middle of the 3 circles and using the answers to the questions, complete the following sentence: *My purpose is…*

Answering these questions may not be easy, and some people may find it useful to mull on them for some time, and possibly even use a trusted and skilled friend or coach to help think it through. But once you have got the answers, it's like a tree having deep roots, helping it to grow and flourish. It may even take several attempts before you feel happy with the result.

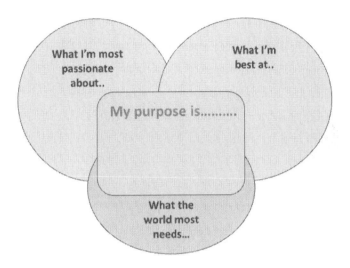

Here's an example from someone who has already done this exercise (and who has agreed we may use their responses in this book):

Stage 1	Write down answers to the questions above and write them into the spaces in each of the circles

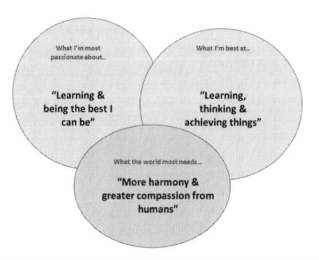

Stage 2	Draw a square in the middle of the 3 circles and using the answers to the questions, complete the following sentence: *My purpose is.....*

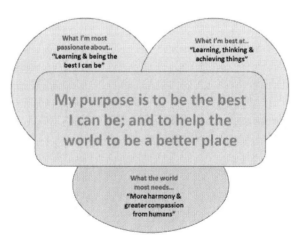

By the end of this exercise, we hope you'll have identified some key drivers in your life. Perhaps you might prefer to describe them as a personal compass, a series of reference points or even a frame. Whatever you decide, this statement can be helpful whenever you feel at a cross roads or need to make some tough decisions. The question to ask yourself is; will this course of action/ decsion/ behaviour take me closer or further away from achieving what I want from my life?

Compassion

The second element of the Happiness Triangle is *compassion,* which is divided into two parts:

- compassion for self
- compassion for others

Compassion for self

How many of us can really say that *we always treat ourselves as we would treat a best friend*? Sadly, the opposite is often true. How many people do you know who work too hard, get excessively stressed, over anxious, depressed, unfit, and involved in bad stuff with other folk, whether family members, work colleagues, neighbours or friends? When it comes to compassion, the very first person we need to learn to show more compassion to, is ourselves – self compassion. A key part of this is first spotting the often unkind things we quietly say to ourselves, and replacing this language with more useful messages. For example, before an important event in your life, you may find your inner critic whispering toxic things in your ears, like: *Typical of you… always late, and never able to do things properly.* When you do spot such unhelpful toxic language in your ear, reject it, and replace it with a new message which you repeat to yourself such as: *Time to show me at my very best. I'm worth it, and I can do it.*

> **Self compassion is the practice of quieting our inner critic, and replacing it with a voice of support, understanding and care for yourself**

Research suggests that self-compassion provides an island of calm, a refuge from the stormy seas of endless positive and negative self-judgment, so that we can finally stop asking, *Am I as good as they are? Am I good enough?* By tapping into our inner wellsprings of kindness, acknowledging the shared nature of our imperfect human condition, we can start to feel more secure, accepted, and alive. It does take work to break the self-criticizing habits of a lifetime, but at the end of the day, you are only being asked to relax, allow life to be as it is, and open your heart to yourself. How to do this? The answer is: *a tiny step each day*: And then, after a surprisingly short time, we can find that a new and positive habit has begun to develop, where we find ourselves beginning to take a bit more care towards our own selves.

Compassion for others

Not surprisingly, the little voice continually chattering away to us also talks about other people and the way we interpret the world around us. Unless we've found a way of saying positive things to ourselves, that voice will probably also say negative things about other people, such as: *She's always late... He's a waste of space... She's a nasty piece of work* or *Typical of him – he never helps out.*

If we stop and listen to ourselves and others, we can sometimes spot and (if we want to) stop the unhelpful self-talk and replace it with something more useful. Most people (us included) do the best they can given the choices we think we have. The thing is, most of us actually have far more choices in how we think and behave than we believe.

Unless we're careful, this internal chatter about ourselves and others can too easily become habits of how we think, and they can, of course, not serve us well – or not so well. By recognizing such unhelpful habits of thinking, we can take the first step towards stopping them and thinking about others in a more helpful and compassionate way.

Every encounter with a person provides us with an opportunity to show a bit of compassion for others. For example, when we're in the checkout queue in the supermarket, the staff member there usually has a name badge on, and the tiniest thing we can do to show more compassion is to call them by their name – a tiny but significant kind act that can make a difference to another person's day. For some reason, most of us hang back from offering feedback to others – even when it's positive. So, another way to show more compassion to others is to look for (genuine) opportunities to say how we enjoy and appreciate certain things others do that affect us.

When we turn our minds to it, there are lots of opportunities to be more generous (in an authentic and sensitive way) with our positive feedback to others.

During the Covid-19 initial lockdown, we've all been touched by many *random acts of kindness* shown all over the world, from Italian people singing from their flat balconies to Brits clapping in the street for NHS and other front-line workers. The Covid-19 period has been a true test of our inner resilience, but as the Mental Health Foundation says:

Doing good makes us feel good

They have more on this on their website at:

https://mentalhealth.org.uk/publications/doing-good-does-you-good

There's a long list of possible random acts of kindness we could easily choose to do, including:

- call a friend we haven't spoken to for a while
- tell a family member how much we love and appreciate them
- make a cup of tea for someone we live with
- arrange to have a cup of tea and virtual catch up with someone we know
- help with an extra household chore at home
- arrange to watch a film at the same time as a friend and video call
- tell someone you know that we are proud of them

- give up our place in the supermarket queue for someone who has only a few items
- calling out thank you when the post comes through the door
- smiling at someone we encounter

The list is endless…

The beauty of seeking to make a random act of kindness each day is that it will not only help someone else, but it will also help ourselves, since the research shows (Dr Stephen Post, 2017) that when we help others, it promotes physiological changes in our brains linked with happiness. As Stephen Post says:

A candle loses nothing of its light by lighting another candle. By lighting the heart of someone else, we allow our own hearts to be lit

It's good to know that Stephen Post is not alone in this thinking. A dynamic and innovative organisation called *kindness.org* believes that kindness is the catalyst for solving the world's greatest challenges. They are a non profit organisation, firmly grounded in quality research, with the mission to educate and inspire people to choose kindness. They encourage people, organisations and communities to take acts of kindness. In so doing, they promote the concept that the accumulation of such acts of kindness has a big impact on building a better world. Their website is: www.kindness.org

They have worked in partnership with Melissa Burmester and Jaclyn Lindsey to publish a book called *Be Kind – A Year of Kindness, One Week at a Time*. The book encourages people to take an act kindness every week for a year, benefitting others, (and therefore themselves), while deepening connections in their communities. In the book, for each of the 52 weeks, there's an inspirational story, some relevant and thought provoking statistics, and suggestions for acts of kindness.

And next, we turn our attention to the third part of the Happiness Triangle, which is *gratitude*.

Gratitude

There's a lot of research which shows the benefits of showing and receiving gratitude, some of which we describe below. From this, we know that the habit of thinking and expressing gratitude has a notable impact on our overall wellbeing. People who practice gratitude experience fewer aches and pains, sleep better, have higher rates of resilience, increased self-esteem, immunity, happiness, energy, optimism, and empathy. A useful place to find out more about this is at:

https://positivepsychology.com/neuroscience-of-gratitude/

From the huge amount of research available, we know when we express and receive gratitude our brain releases dopamine and serotonin, the two crucial neurotransmitters responsible for our emotions. They enhance our mood immediately, making us feel happy from the inside. By consciously practicing gratitude every day, we can help these neural pathways to strengthen themselves and ultimately create a permanent grateful and positive nature within ourselves. The effect of gratitude on the brain is long lasting (Moll, Zahn, et al. 2007). Besides enhancing self-love and empathy, gratitude significantly impacts on body functions and psychological conditions like stress, anxiety, and depression. Gratitude gets rid of toxic emotions in our bodies.

A study called *Counting Blessings vs Burdens* (2003) evaluated the effect of gratitude on physical well-being. It concluded that sixteen percent of the participants who kept a gratitude journal reported better physical health. Another research study (Zahn et al., 2009) showed that showing gratitude improves sleep quality. This study showed that a brain filled with gratitude and kindness is more likely to sleep better and wake up feeling refreshed and energetic every morning.

Finally, we now also know that gratitude helps us to manage our stress and anxiety levels. McCraty and colleagues (1998), in one of their studies on gratitude and appreciation, found that participants who felt grateful showed a marked reduction in the level of cortisol, the stress hormone. They had better cardiac functioning and were more resilient to emotional setbacks and negative experiences. Significant studies over the years have established the fact that by practicing gratitude we can handle stress better than others. By merely acknowledging and appreciating the little things in life, we can rewire the brain to deal with the present circumstances with more awareness and broader perception.

All well and good, but how, in the real world, can we go about this? Below are some ideas:

- each day, (or night), reflect on any good thing that's happened over the past day. This can be as simple as enjoying a decent cup of coffee, reading a joke or finding a car parking space on a busy Friday morning.
- write *gratitude letters*. A gratitude letter is written to someone in your life to express appreciation for ways they have helped you and/or been there for you. Gratitude letters can be about events that have happened in the past or are happening in the present, and often help to strengthen or repair relationships.
- make a gratitude list. A gratitude list involves writing down three to five things for which we're grateful every day, each week, at other intervals, or under situation-specific circumstances.

Action for Happiness

Before we end this chapter on happiness, it's important to applaud the work of the Action for Happiness movement. *Action for Happiness* was co-founded in 2010 by Richard Layard, (Director of the Wellbeing Programme at the Centre for Economic Performance and Emeritus Professor of Economics at LSE), Sir Anthony Seldon (Historian and Vice-

Chancellor of the University of Buckingham), amongst others. They describe happiness thus:

> *Happiness means feeling good about our lives and wanting to go on feeling that way. Unhappiness means feeling bad and wanting things to change*
>
> (Layard 2020)

The *Action for Happiness* organisation supports people to understand that everybody has an inner world and mental health, and that everybody can choose to take action to look after their mental health, in good times as well as bad times. Just like choosing to look after our physical health by exercising and eating good food, we can look after our mind by developing skills to be happy.

They promote *Ten Keys to Happier Living* which are based on the latest research in positive psychology, neuroscience, behavioural economics and biology. Their research evidence suggests these Ten Keys, once embedded into our lives, can have a significant and positive impact on our happiness and well-being. The Ten Keys are spelled out as GREAT DREAM. The first five keys (GREAT) are about our interaction with the outside world. The second five keys (DREAM) relate to our inner world and depend on our attitude to life.

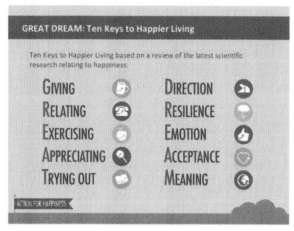

<u>Action For Happiness</u>[ii]

G IVING   Do things for others

Caring about others is fundamental to our happiness. Helping other people is not only good for them and a great thing to do, it also makes us happier and healthier too. Giving also creates stronger connections between people and helps to build a happier society for everyone. And it's not all about money - we can also give our time, ideas and energy. So if we want to feel good, do good!

R ELATING   Connect with people

Relationships are the most important overall contributor to happiness. People with strong and broad social relationships are happier, healthier and live longer. Close relationships with family and friends provide love, meaning, support and increase our feelings of self worth. Broader networks bring a sense of belonging. So taking action to strengthen our relationships and create new connections is essential for happiness.

E XERCISING   Take care of our body

Our body and our mind are connected. Being active makes us happier as well as being good for our physical health. It instantly improves our mood and can even lift us out of a depression. We don't all need to run marathons – there are simple things we can all do to be more active each day. We can also boost our well-being by unplugging from technology, getting outside and making sure we get enough sleep.

A WARENESS   Live life mindfully

Ever felt there must be more to life? Well good news, there is. And it's right here in front of us. We just need to stop and take notice. Learning to be more mindful and aware does wonders for our well-being in all areas of life – like our walk to work, the way we eat or our relationships. It helps us get in tune with our feelings and stops us dwelling on the past or worrying about the future – so we get more out of the day-to-day.

T RYING OUT   Keep learning new things

Learning affects our well-being in lots of positive ways. It exposes us to new ideas and helps us stay curious and engaged. It also gives us a sense of accomplishment and helps boost our self-confidence and resilience. There are many ways to learn new things – not just through formal qualifications. We can share a skill with friends, join a club, learn to sing, play a new sport and so much more.

D IRECTION Have goals to look forward to

Feeling good about the future is important for our happiness. We all need goals to motivate us and these need to be challenging enough to excite us, but also achievable. If we try to attempt the impossible this brings unnecessary stress. Choosing ambitious but realistic goals gives our lives direction and brings a sense of accomplishment and satisfaction when we achieve them.

R ESILIENCE Find ways to bounce back

All of us have times of stress, loss, failure or trauma in our lives. But how we respond to these has a big impact on our well-being. We often cannot choose what happens to us, but we can choose our own attitude to what happens. In practice it's not always easy, but one of the most exciting findings from recent research is that resilience, like many other life skills, can be learned.

E MOTIONS Focus on what's good

Positive emotions – like joy, gratitude, contentment, inspiration, and pride – are not just great at the time. Regularly experiencing them creates an upward spiral, helping to build our resources. So, although we need to be realistic about life's ups and downs, it helps to focus on the good aspects of any situation – the glass half full rather than the glass half empty.

A CCEPTANCE Be comfortable with who we are

No-one's perfect. But so often we compare our insides to other people's outsides. Dwelling on our flaws – what we're not rather than what we've got – makes it much harder to be happy. Learning to accept ourselves, warts and all, and being kinder to ourselves when things go wrong, increases our enjoyment of life, our resilience and our well-being. It also helps us accept others as they are.

M EANING Be part of something bigger

People who have meaning and purpose in their lives are happier, feel more in control and get more out of what they do. They also experience less stress, anxiety and depression. But where do we find meaning and purpose? It might be our religious faith, being a parent or doing a job that makes a difference. The answers vary for each of us but they all involve being connected to something bigger than ourselves.

You can find out more about the Action for Happiness movement by accessing this link:

https://www.actionforhappiness.org/

They have local networks, each of which run a range of courses and support to enable people to continue to learn and develop.

Bad stuff will happen to all of us, at some time, but the more we are happy, deep down, the more resilient we will be to bounce back from adversity and to help others do the same.

Here's a saying we've always found useful. It dates back to Epictetus, a Greek philosopher who lived in the first century:

> *It's not what happens to you, but how you react to it that matters. When something happens, the only thing in your power is your attitude toward it; you can either accept it or resent it*

To sum up, in this chapter we've considered the very foundations of happiness:

- having a sense of purpose in our lives
- showing compassion to ourselves and to others
- experiencing and expressing gratitude

These three very special aspects of life make up the first Tool in our Happiness Toolkit:

1. Purpose, compassion & gratitude

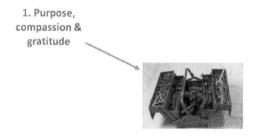

Happiness Toolkit

However, to get to a position where we can think, talk and write about such things requires another set of skills: *awareness of self and others* - which we explore more in the next chapter.

Chapter two: Developing awareness

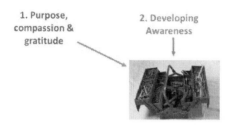

Happiness Toolkit

In this chapter, we explore the second Tool in our Happiness Toolkit: how our awareness of self and others lays the foundation for our happiness. In particular, we'll be exploring the need, on occasions, for us to:

- adopt different perspectives in how we see things
- reframe how we think about things
- practise mindfulness

Most people, if asked the question: *Are you self-aware?* would probably say: *Of course I am* and this is no doubt true, up to a point. What's interesting is that there's a wide range of self-awareness available to all of us and we all fit somewhere on that range. Another question might be: *Could you be even more self-aware?* Most people, reading this book at least, would probably say yes to that question. The trouble is the majority of our thoughts, feelings and actions are driven by habit or autopilot. (That's why, for example, we sometimes find ourselves wondering if we've locked the door once we've left the house). It's useful to have so many things driven by habit. Our automated habits and routines help us in our lives so we don't have to stop and think every time we leave the house or go to start the car.

The problem arises when we're on autopilot for so long that we forget we're on autopilot and we're not even aware of our own habits and routines. In that scenario they control us, whereas a person with self-awareness is able to exercise a little of that self-awareness and say, *Hmm... every time my sister calls me and asks for money, I end up drinking a lot more than I should. That might not be a coincidence.* A person without this level of self-awareness remains stuck in the pattern of behaviour.

We need at this stage to define our terms a bit more clearly. What is self-awareness? Paul Silvia and Maureen O'Brien (2004) define it as *the capacity to focus attention on oneself and to self-evaluate.*

For us, the critical and often the most challenging aspect of this is *self-evaluation*. This requires us to be open to the idea that how others see the world is not necessarily the same as we see it. Thus, self-awareness and self-evaluation require the skill of understanding self and self in relation to others. Why is self-awareness so important?

- with greater self-awareness, we see life differently and more thoroughly

More awareness allows us to view life through various lenses, perspectives, and possibilities. It embodies the opportunities to evaluate what should change, what new habits need to be formed, and the ultimate dreams we really do have for our life: these things will push us to achieve goals previously only dreamt about.

- with greater self-awareness, we better understand the world around us

Along with seeing our life differently, more awareness enables us to see others and the world around us differently. We process different emotions, scenarios, and experiences through a healthy filter. We become a more understanding and nicer person. A better understanding gives us more space to be gentler on our self and others. As new habits begin to form, we start automatically choosing to see the positives in more things. This new perspective ultimately leads to a journey towards happiness.

- with greater self-awareness, we manage our inner world much better

With more awareness in place, our attitude and perspective become clearer over time. The more we practice and embrace awareness, the more our perspective will shift. With a clearer perspective, we process things better. We see the good around us and don't dwell on the negative. Happiness doesn't just happen, it's chosen. By choosing more awareness, we can find an inner peace with what happens in life.

The following story illustrates how each person's awareness is constrained and shaped by what we each can see and experience – and how far removed our awareness often is from how things *really* are:

A long ago, six old men lived in a village in India. Each was born blind. The other villagers loved the old men and kept them away from harm. Since the blind men could not see the world for themselves, they had to imagine many of its wonders. The old men had heard about elephants but of course had never seen one. They asked the Rajah to take them to an elephant so they could find out what it was like. The Rajah's servant led them to a courtyard where there stood an elephant. The blind men stepped forward to touch the great creature. The first blind man reached out and touched the side of the huge animal.

"An elephant is smooth and solid like a wall!" he declared.

The second blind man put his hand on the elephant's trunk. "An elephant is like a giant snake," he announced.

The third blind man felt the elephant's pointed tusk. "This creature is as sharp and deadly as a spear."

The fourth blind man touched one of the elephant's four legs. "What we have here," he said, "is an extremely large cow."

The fifth blind man felt the elephant's giant ear. "I believe an elephant is like a huge fan or maybe a magic carpet that can fly over mountains and treetops," he said.

The sixth blind man gave a tug on the elephant's coarse tail. "Why, this is nothing more than a piece of old rope. Dangerous, indeed," he scoffed.

The six blind men then went and sat under a tree and argued furiously about what an elephant is like.

"An elephant is like a wall," said the first blind man. "Surely we can finally agree on that."

"A wall? An elephant is a giant snake!"

"It's a spear, I tell you."

"I'm certain it's a giant cow."

"Magic carpet. There's no doubt."

"Don't you see? Someone used a rope to trick us."

Their argument continued and their shouts grew louder and louder.

"Wall!"

"Snake!"

"Spear!"

"Cow!"

"Carpet!"

"Rope!"

"Stop shouting!" called a very angry voice.

It was the Rajah, awakened from his nap by the noisy argument.

"How can each of you be so certain you are right?" asked the ruler.

The six blind men considered the question.

"The elephant is a very large animal," said the Rajah kindly. "Each man touched only one part. Perhaps if you put the parts together, you will see the truth. Now, let me finish my nap in peace."

After a while, once they had pondered on the Rajah's advice, the first blind man sighed and simply said:

"He is right. To learn the truth, we must put all the parts together. Let's discuss this on the journey home."

This story goes to the heart of an old expression by Alfred Korzybski (1933):

The map is not the territory

In the rest of this chapter, we'll explore how more awareness can help us to understand different perspectives. Understanding this point is a key part of living a life in harmony with others and is fundamental to living a happier life.

None of us see the world as it is. We create and use our own map of the world, which is different from the reality of the world and different from other people's maps. We're now going on to explore three specific aspects of this:

- experiencing the world from different perspectives
- the skill of reframing
- the importance of mindfulness

Experiencing the world from different perspectives

Before you criticise a man, walk a mile in his moccasins is a Native American saying which neatly illustrates this concept. The implication here is the importance of understanding at least three different perspectives; our own, that of another person and of someone who is an observer to whatever is taking place – sometimes called *perceptual positions. (Bandler and Grinder 1987).*

Perceptual positions

Perceptual positions is a way of seeing things from a number of perspectives, and thus giving us a richer understanding of a situation. The three main perspectives include:

- first position – seeing something through our own eyes
- second position – seeing something through the eyes of others
- third position – seeing things as if we are a fly on the wall - a neutral observer

The more we can practise the skill of seeing things through all of these positions, the more we will be able to understand an issue or situation; and the more we do this, the more we can make better choices about how to respond.

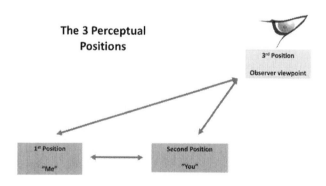

First position

When we're in first position, our attention is on our own feelings, needs and goals, to the neglect of the other person. We are aware of our own concerns but relatively blind to the concerns of the other person.

Second position

When we're in second position, we see the world (as much as we can) from the other person's perspective. Our attention is on the other person's feelings, needs and goals, and the effect of what we say and do on that person. We're more aware of (what we think are) their concerns than of our own. Psychologically we are where they are: which in turn helps us understand them, and how they think. As Gregory Bateson (1972) said:

> *If you want to understand something, you have to think about it the way that thing thunk*

Third position

When we're in third position, we're an observer to the whole situation. Our attention is on the interaction between self and the other people involved in a situation. We're a disinterested observer, aware of the nature of the exchange between self and this other person. Psychologically we're a fly on the wall. Third position is useful when we want to shift from emotionally charged experiences to get an objective view.

Third position is useful for stepping back and getting insights into situations and seeing and hearing the bigger picture.

So, how, in the real world, can we use these different perspectives, in a way that's helpful?

Imagine this scenario:

Someone comes to us in distress, saying;

I've had another terrible day at work… another argument with my workmate. He's such a toad, I hate him. I can't go on like this.

We have the advantage of knowing there is no single way of seeing situations, and we suspect our friend is only seeing the position from *first position,* i.e. their own viewpoint.

Here are some suggestions about what we might want to do:

Listen well

First of all, listen even more to your friend… allowing them to be heard and possibly even coming to their own solution.

Ask questions to understand their viewpoint (their first position)

Then, ask them questions to make sure we understand fully why this matters to them.

Ask questions to explore the situation from the other person's viewpoint (i.e. second position):

- *Help me understand this from your workmate's perspective*
- *What do you think is going on with your workmate right now?*
- *What pressures do you think your workmate is feeling right now?*
- *Tell me about other times when your workmate has responded better*
- *If you were in your workmate's shoes, how would you be feeling and what would you be wanting to do instead?*

Ask questions from the perspective of a neutral observer, (i.e. third position):

- *If you were a fly on the wall, what would you be noticing about what's going on between you and your workmate?*
- *Staying as a fly on the wall for a moment longer, what patterns are you now noticing that you may not have spotted before?*

Finally, we might want to suggest that we go for a walk or share a cup of tea or coffee, when we can encourage them to reflect on everything that's been said, and explore how these different perspectives change and how they will respond in future. Hopefully, this intervention will have helped them to see the situation in a different light and have more ideas about how to respond better in the future.

Seeing things in a different light, and thus realising we have more and better options in dealing situations is a key skill, which is sometimes called *reframing* and that's where we're going next.

The skill of reframing

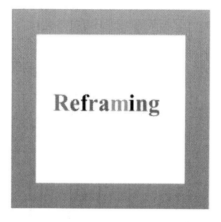

Reframing is the second way to increase the perspectives we use to see the world. It's an invaluable technique of being able to change the frame we put round things; and the exact frame we use can have a dramatic difference to how we think about the issue. The classic reframe that we all know is when we see a partly consumed beer glass, is it half full or half empty? There's probably a well rooted belief in our culture that our thoughts can't, don't or won't change. Have you ever heard someone say *That's me. Take it or leave it.* They are mistaken. The more self-aware we are, the more we know that we can, to an extent, choose or modify how we think about things, especially using this technique of changing the frame we use around our thoughts, i.e. reframing.

Frames are a major part of the system of filters through which we represent things internally. They act as mental templates or patterns, through which we experience the world. The frame we set, consciously or unconsciously, reflects the way we perceive things or the way we look at them. *Reframing* means changing the frame of reference around a behaviour, statement or event, finding another meaning or interpretation, seeing things in a different light. Often, we can find ourselves stuck in the rut of certain ways of thinking – our fixed mindsets, resulting sometimes in us missing out on new ways of solving problems or understanding what's going on.

Here's an example of how, if we change the frame through which we interpret things, we change the meaning. The same picture – two different frames; and vastly different interpretations:

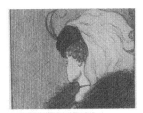

Beautiful young lady, looking away from you

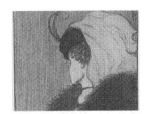

Old lady with a hooked nose looking down and sad

My Wife and my Mother-in-law[iii]

If we get a knock on the door at midday we might welcome it, possibly expecting a parcel to arrive. If the same thing happens at midnight when we're in bed, our response will probably be different, and we might get alarmed. Same event, different frame, and therefore a different response. Much of comedy is based on reframes: a sudden new way of seeing things. For example, one of the classic comedy reframes is probably Eric Morecombe's *I'm playing the right notes – but not necessarily in the right order.*

A useful example of reframing is the often uttered comment:

In the big scheme of things, how important is this?

This simple question has the power to change significantly a huge issue into something which is not so important because we're being invited to see it in a larger context. i.e. a different frame.

We explore in chapter seven the common human behaviour of using negative self-talk about ourselves, such as:

- *I'm not good enough*
- *I'm a failure*
- *I feel helpless*

Once we have, hopefully, stopped such negative self-talk in its tracks, we can use reframing to change such thoughts. For example, imagine someone says to themselves something like:

Rainy days make me feel depressed. I hate rainy days.

Imagine thinking that every half hour or so throughout the course of a rainy day! There are lots of possible ways to reframe such thinking, including:

Ah, good, another day for staying inside all day, all snug and safe, and able to do one of my passions which is my craft work.

or…

Another chance to get all dressed up and warm and go for a walk in the woods.

Let's say someone we know has a habit of running down other people we care about. How might we reframe the situation?

- he's feeling ill
- he didn't get a good night's sleep
- he's stressed about something
- other people treat him in the same way
- he suffered abuse as a child
- he has a terminal illness

A key skill in living a happy and productive life is the ability to be aware of the frames we use to make sense of the world around us and, if appropriate, to make better choices of these frames.

The third element of seeing things through different perspectives is mindfulness.

Mindfulness

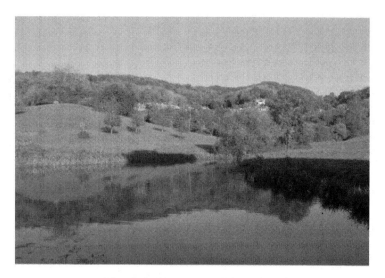

Mind full or Mindful?

It can be easy to rush through life without stopping to notice much. Paying more attention to the present moment – to our own thoughts and feelings, and to the world around us – can improve our mental wellbeing. Some people call this *mindfulness*. Mindfulness can help us enjoy life more and understand ourselves better. It's also incredibly powerful in helping us become more self-aware. What is mindfulness? On his website, Professor Mark Williams, former director of the Oxford Mindfulness Centre, (www.psych.ox.ac.uk) says that mindfulness means knowing directly what is going on inside and outside ourselves, moment by moment.

It's easy to stop noticing the world around us. It's also easy to lose touch with the way our bodies are feeling and to end up living in our heads, caught up in our thoughts without stopping to notice how those thoughts are driving our emotions and behaviour. An important part of mindfulness is reconnecting with our bodies and the sensations they experience. This means waking up to the sights, sounds, smells and tastes of the present moment. That might be something as simple as the feel of a banister as we walk upstairs. A second important part of mindfulness is an awareness of our thoughts and feelings as they happen moment to moment. It's about allowing ourselves to see the present moment clearly.

When we do that, it can positively change the way we see ourselves and our lives and enhance our wellbeing. Becoming more aware of the present moment can help us enjoy the world around us more and understand ourselves better. When we become more aware of the present moment, we begin to experience afresh things that we have been taking for granted. As Professor Williams writes:

> *Mindfulness also allows us to become more aware of the stream of thoughts and feelings that we experience and to see how we can become entangled in that stream in ways that are not helpful*

Gradually, we can train ourselves to notice when our thoughts are taking over and realise that thoughts are simply mental events that do not have to control us. Most of us have issues that we find hard to let go and mindfulness can help us deal with them more productively. We can ask: *Is trying to solve this by brooding about it helpful, or am I just getting caught up in my thoughts?*

Awareness of this kind also helps us notice signs of stress or anxiety earlier and helps us deal with them better. Mindfulness is recommended by the National Institute for Health and Care Excellence (NICE) as a way to prevent depression in people who have had three or more bouts of depression in the past. So how does anyone become more mindful? There is advice from the NHS, blogs, courses to attend and YouTube clips but here, we've drawn up some simple steps to begin personal practice.

Notice what's going on inside	Reminding our self to take notice of thoughts, feelings, body sensations and the world around us. This is the first step to mindfulness.
	Professor Williams writes:
	Even as we go about our daily lives, we can notice the sensations of things, the food we eat, the air moving past the body as we walk. All this may sound very small, but it has huge power to interrupt the 'autopilot' mode we often engage day to

	day, and to give us new perspectives on life
Keep it regular	It can be helpful to pick a regular time – the morning journey to work or a walk at lunchtime – when we decide to be especially aware of the sensations created by the world around us
Try something new	Trying new things, such as sitting in a different seat in meetings or going somewhere new for lunch, can also help us notice the world in a new way
Free yourself from the past and future	Left to its own devices, the human brain tends to dwell on thoughts about the past, or to fixate on thoughts about the future. We need to notice such patterns in our own thinking and say something quietly about being more interested in the now

	rather than being trapped in the past, or pre-living the future
Name some of your thoughts and feelings	To develop an awareness of thoughts and feelings Some people find it helpful to name them. Instead of worrying that we might fail that exam, name it. For example: *I'm feeling anxious about that exam*
Watch your thoughts	Many people find it difficult to practice, largely because of the inevitable intrusion of lots of thoughts and worries that often come into our heads. Mindfulness isn't about stopping these thoughts, but rather as seeing them in a different way. For example, imagine standing at a bus station and seeing a stream of *thought buses* coming and going, without having to get on the buses and being taken away by them.

	Some people also find it easier to cope with an over busy mind if they do gentle yoga or walking

Mindfulness meditation involves sitting silently and paying attention to thoughts, sounds, the sensations of breathing or parts of the body, bringing attention back whenever the mind starts to wander. Yoga and tai chi can also help with developing awareness of our thinking and breathing.

Further useful advice on mindfulness can be found in lots of places, including the following NHS internet site:

https://www.nhs.uk/conditions/stress-anxiety-depression/mindfulness/

So far in this book, we've explored the following first 2 Tools in our Happiness Toolbox:

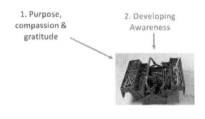

Happiness Toolkit

Soon, we'll be moving onto the third Tool, which is *Taking Actions*. But first, we need to focus on *Where to Start?*

Chapter three: Where to start?

Does anyone ever wake up in the morning and say, *Right, this is what I'm going to do in my life from now on?* Bingo, they have the perfect scenario for achieving their goals and dreams? No.

Yes, well perhaps some people might say this is what happened but we're sure there's probably been a lot of soul searching, a lot of wakeful nights and time spent either alone or with a trusted ally or two when ideas have tumbled out. Most of the time, many people have a feeling that translates into words such as *Life sucks* or *I'm at a dead end in my career/ love life/ health/ weight...* please feel free to fill in as many blanks as you can. In our experience, most of us often reach a point when we know something must change. Perhaps there's been a trigger, a big birthday, watching your children toddle off to university, the death of a parent and now we're the older generation, realising time is finite and those closest to us are settling down, getting onto the career ladder, moving away or simply moving on.

When that moment arrives, we often recognise it's time to take some action.

Except where do we start?

For many years now we've done a Life Audit on a regular basis. There are many different ways you can approach this but one thing we ask is that you use pen and paper. *Think in ink* is the phrase we often use. Moon (2006) identifies learning as taking place as a result of writing through the process of slowing the learning process down, forcing the writer to organize their thoughts and helping to clarify the issue. We would go even further and suggest that using language to describe what may only be a vague sensation enables the learner to interact with the sensation. Giving it a concrete form means that it can be managed both by the individual and shared with others.

To do this, we suggest being creative with colours or types of paper. But how you go about this is *your* decision. It's time to take real ownership of the process we will take you through. All we ask is that you *write*, not type your responses.

So, pen in hand, make a list as long as you like of any topics in your life at the moment.

Here's a starter:

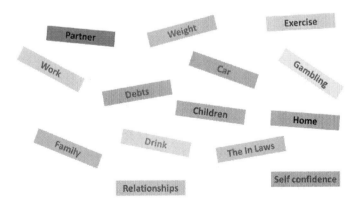

You might want to be more specific. For example:

Weight:

I used to be at my ideal weight for years. Now I'm carrying fifteen pounds too much. I hate it. My arms are flabby and I've got the start of a double chin

Money:

I'm maxed out on my credit cards and have bills coming in next week. I don't like living from month to month. I'm always struggling

Work:

I'm in a dead end job. The boss is an idiot. My co workers are great

Partner:

We're going through the motions. We argue all the time

Another, more structured way of identify the areas to work on is to use a Life Audit, as below:

Life Audit: currently:

If I had more time, I would:
I resent time spent on:
I love spending time on:
My regrets:
My wishes:

Life Audit: my new and ideal future:

My top priorities in life:

My most important values in life:

Specific outcomes I intend to achieve in the next 12 months:

What would make me happiest in the next 12 months:

Take your time over this, as it forms the basis for everything else that follows.

When you've got an exhaustive list, you may find the items can be grouped into categories, e.g. health, career, relationships.

TOPIC	THEMES
WORK	I was overlooked for promotion The boss is always on at me I'm bored and I know I can do more This job is going nowhere I dread Monday I worry I'm not going to be able to keep to all my deadlines
HOME	My place is a mess. I've read all the stuff about decluttering but I can't do it The place needs redecorating. I can't afford to get anyone in and I'm sure to make a mess of it. Where do I start? Everyone else has a nice home
PARTNER	We argue over little things He won't talk to me She doesn't listen when I say we need to spend less I can't trust him She puts her friends before me. Why can't we spend some time just chilling out together? Why does she always want to go shopping? I think he/she is seeing someone else We never kiss and cuddle. It's always sex

SELF CONFIDENCE	Why can't I stand up for myself when the boss dumps more work on me? I feel a failure I feel ugly and unloved and unlovable. If I was more confident, it'd be great I'm frightened for the future

And so on…We're sure you can continue with this as it's a bit of a blurt or a rant about what's wrong with your life. And it's okay. Getting this onto paper, in language, is the first step to change. It might be that already you have identified an area you felt was a problem and now it isn't, once it's been put into words on paper. Sometimes that's enough.

If not, we can move onto the next step which is about scaling.

Have you ever heard the phrase *On a scale of one to ten* or *On a scale from one to five?* Perhaps you've given feedback on a restaurant or a hotel and used a star rating? Such things are used a lot. Your task now is to give each of these areas a rating too. We use a rating of one to ten where ten is perfect and zero is… awful. There's a rationale behind this system of rating. It's based on the work of a psychologist called Rensis Likert who developed a five and a seven-point scale. We suggest a ten-point scale as it gives us slightly more flexibility. Is it valid to self-rate like this? Well, yes as research has shown we are perfectly capable of assessing ourselves over time and individuals can also be very aware of their own skills and strengths (Rajecki, 1990).

For each area you have identified, please give it a score from one to ten. It might end up something like this:

TOPIC	THEMES
HEALTH AND FITNESS 5/10	Weight: I used to be at my ideal weight for years. Now I'm carrying fifteen pounds too much. I hate it. My arms are flabby and I've got the start of a double chin I'm not as fit as I'd like. I can't run after the grandkids in the park I'm flabby I can't sleep at night and I'm always tired
WORK 5/10	I was overlooked for promotion The boss is always on at me I'm bored and I know I can do more This job is going nowhere I dread Monday I worry I'm not going to be able to keep to all my deadlines
HOME 7/10	My place is a mess. I've read all the stuff about decluttering but I can't do it

	The place needs redecorating. I can't afford to get anyone in and I'm sure to make a mess of it. Where do I start? Everyone else has a nice home
PARTNER 3/10	We argue over little things He won't talk to me She doesn't listen when I say we need to spend less I can't trust him She puts her friends before me. Why can't we spend some time just chilling out together? Why does she always want to go shopping? I think he/she is seeing someone else. We never kiss and cuddle. It's always sex
SELF CONFIDENCE 1/10	Why can't I stand up for myself when the boss dumps more work on me? I feel a failure I feel ugly and unloved and unlovable. If I was more confident, it'd be great I'm frightened for the future

What then? It's time to decide which three areas you would like to work on.

Why three? Check out what it says on the power of three in an internet search. From numerology to religion, marketing to popular stories (Three Blind Mice, Goldilocks and the Three Bears etc.), the number three often recurs. And there's a good reason for this; it seems the brain remembers three things more easily than anything else so selecting three areas to work on gives our brain a better chance to remember, retain and handle.

Got your three areas? Good: because now's the time to do something about them.

Chapter four: How to make this happen

Action plans? Project management? Plan, Do Review? Target setting? Yes, we've all heard of them. Some of us are more familiar with action planning and workstreams than with a recipe book. They're as much a part of working life as Monday morning. We can adopt the best parts as we begin to take action on our three key areas.

Most workplaces will have used SMART targets or goals, either for team projects, individual performance management or outcomes for the next few months. As a reminder, these are the meanings:

S	Specific. State what you'll do. Use action words
M	Measurable. Make you know how to measure your success & outcomes
A	Achievable. Make sure your actions are in your control to do; and it's possible to do them
R	Realistic. Check out that the actions are possible; & assess & plans for risks
T	Timebound. Give deadlines for the action & outcomes

These are great as a starter but over the past few years we've adopted a variant on this which has come from the school of thought called NLP (Neuro Linguistic Programming), devised originally by Richard Bandler and John Grinder. It was popular in the later decades of the last century and in the early years of the 21st century and is still going strong today with conferences, training programmes and master classes.

Through NLP we came across the *well-formed outcome* which has some elements of SMART targets but goes a little bit further in identifying what might sabotage achieving any target or goal. To create a goal or as we will call it from now on, an outcome, it has to satisfy these criteria:

LETTER	WHAT DOES THIS MEAN?	EXPLANATION	EXAMPLE
P	Positive	Any outcome needs to be in positive language	I want a tidy house. I want more self confidence
E	Ecology	Do I really want this goal? If there is any hesitation, that needs to be explored in more detail	Yes. Of course
S	Specific	When do I want this to happen?	I want a tidy house before the end of

			this coming month
E	Evidence	What will I see? Hear? (What will that little voice inside my head be saying?) Feel?	Everything will be cleared away or in its place. I'll be hearing myself say 'Wow that is great' and I'll feel a real sense of achievement
O	Own control	Is this in my own power to achieve?	Yes. Providing I get going and don't sit around wishing it would happen

The O for OWN CONTROL needs a bit of clarification. We are only in control of ourselves. Yes, we may want the boss to recognise our worth and give us that post we want. We cannot control his/her responses. What is in our control is to do the best job we can, make sure we apply for any posts we think are appropriate and be personable which includes being reliable, pleasant and kind. No one wants a miserable, unreliable, moaning co-worker who sees life through an embittered, resentful lens. You may still not get the promotion but that may mean you have to go elsewhere and that choice is within your own control. In fact, the choice about how you present yourself on a daily basis *is* within your choice. There will be more about that in a later chapter. For the purpose of this exercise, it's important to recognise your part in achieving any outcome.

As a contrast, here's an example that does *not* meet the criteria and is heading for failure and is still using the tidy house outcome.

LETTER	WHAT DOES THIS MEAN?	EXPLANATION	EXAMPLE
P	Positive	Any outcome needs to be in positive language.	*I don't want a messy house*
E	Ecology	Do I really want this goal? If there is any hesitation, that needs to be explored in more detail	*I suppose so*

S	Specific	When do I want this to happen?	*Any time soon*
E	Evidence	What will I see? Hear? (What will that little voice inside my head be saying?) Feel?	*It won't be a mess anymore*
O	Own outcome	Is this in my own power to achieve?	*If the kids and my partner take their share too*

Here's the same model, shown as a diagram:

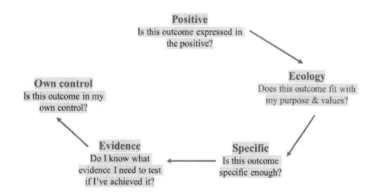

You might have noticed something about the section called *Ecology*. If you find yourself answering in a less than an enthusiastic way about achieving your outcome, ask yourself this question:

What's stopping me from wanting this?

There might be a number of reasons e.g.:

Will it take up too much time? What will other people think? Will I be upsetting anyone?
Is it something I really want or am I feeling pressured?

The answer to these questions will help. For example, it may be a concern over time and you find yourself saying *Yes, I want a tidy home but not if it means I have to spend all my spare time on housework. I want time for me too.*

That's a clear indication that your outcome statement *I want a tidy house* might need to be accompanied by the qualifier, *providing I still have some free time for me.*

You may need to go through this loop several times until you can answer the question, *If you could have this goal now, would you take it?* with a resounding *Yes!* Otherwise there might still be something that will hold you back and sabotage any chances of success.

Here are some examples of outcomes that regularly flounder on the ecology check and a possible resolution.

OUTCOME	RESERVATIONS	NEW OUTCOME
I want promotion	Will it impact on the amount of time I get to spend with the family?	I want promotion and have a work life balance
I want to be a healthy weight.	Do I have to give up all the food I like?	I want to be a healthy weight and still enjoy the food I eat
I want to start saving for my future.	I don't want to appear a mean person	I want to start saving for my future and still be able to treat friends and family and myself from time to time

If you find this a bit of a struggle, try completing the following table using some of all of the questions as prompts.

	QUESTIONS TO ASK	ANSWERS
1	So what is the first area that I want to work on?	
2	What's the problem?	

3	What would I prefer to have? What would I prefer? What would I like to have instead? What would I prefer to feel/think?	
4	If I could get this issue sorted TODAY, would I be okay with that? Is this something I REALLY want?	
5	If not, what else is making things complicated? What needs to be different? What's holding me back from saying 'Yes, I want this now?' AT THIS POINT YOU MAY WANT TO REPEAT QUESTION 4 UNTIL YOU GET A POSITIVE RESPONSE	
6	When do I want this issue to be solved? When do I want to achieve this goal?	

	When do I want this to happen?	
7	How will I know I've achieved this goal? What evidence will I get when I have achieved this goal? What will I see? What will I hear? What will I feel? Is there any other evidence?	
8	Is achieving this goal in my own control?	

It's really worthwhile spending time on this section as it is the basis for what comes next which is to start *taking actions.*

Chapter five: Taking actions

We're now ready to focus on the third Tool in our Happiness Toolkit, which is *Taking Actions.*

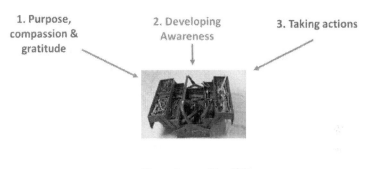

| 1. Purpose, compassion & gratitude | 2. Developing Awareness | 3. Taking actions |

Happiness Toolkit

By the time you reach this stage, we hope you're fired up to take action. Although is that the problem? Is your history peppered with new starts, unfulfilled New Year's Resolutions and so many occasions when you have said to yourself: *This time it's going to be different?*

Be reassured, you're not alone. As far as New Year's Resolutions go, it's estimated only eight percent of Americans who make a New Year's resolution keep them all year. And as many as eighty percent have failed by the start of February. Furthermore, research suggests that one reason resolutions fail is because they're not specific enough. We've already nailed that one. Our action plans are designed not to fall into that trap. But there are other comments from researchers suggesting that we fail because we lack discipline or we self sabotage. We'll come back to that in a later chapter. For the moment, it's time to start taking small steps to achieve our outcomes.

So what will those small steps be? It may be that you say, *I don't know what to do or how to do it.* That's fine. There are loads of internet sites you can search for ideas about changing diet, getting healthy, feeling more confident, or getting that dream job. For example, when we searched on *Overcoming Loneliness,* there was a huge amount of good ideas, information, contacts, facts, figures, not to mention videos from people who have been in a similar situation.

One of the pieces of advice we've learnt is to make sure any steps are small enough to achieve. For example, how many people have you come across who decide to get fit as from the first of January They join a gym, hit the roads for a morning jog and it lasts three weeks as they end up exhausted and perhaps even with an injury that puts paid to their plans. Why? Too much too soon. It's far better to join the gym and go once for the first few weeks, after you've had a session with one of the personal trainers to devise a schedule for your individual needs. That should come free with your membership. If your aim is to run at seven mph on the treadmill for twenty minutes, the first week, you might set yourself a walk at four mph for five minutes and increase only when you feel comfortable. Our suggestion is to take small steps and celebrate each and every achievement, however small. You'll deserve it.

We've drawn up a possible format to help you to keep this in mind.

GOAL/ OUTCOME		
DATES	**ACTION/ACTIONS**	**EVIDENCE IT'S BEEN ACHIEVED**
WEEK ONE	1. 2. 3. 4.	
WEEK TWO		
WEEK THREE		
WEEK FOUR		
RESULTS SO FAR AND CELEBRATION		

We've populated one table with fitness as an example:

GOAL/ OUTCOME:
To be able to complete a 5K charity race on October 15th 2021

DATES	ACTION/ACTIONS	EVIDENCE IT'S BEEN ACHIEVED AND DATE
WEEK ONE	1.Join gym 2. Meet with coach, Graham and agree on a routine 3. Begin one session of routine 4. Walk to shops on Saturday	2 April 4 April 4 April 6 April despite rain!
WEEK TWO	1.Session 2 of routine 2. Increase speed on treadmill by 0.5 3. Get off bus one stop earlier each working day 4. Session 3 in gym. Maintain speed	9 April Up to 4.5 mph Yes: could I save some money? 4.5 but also did two minutes at 4.5
WEEK THREE	1.Session 4 of routine 2. Maintain speed, increase time by two minutes 3. Session 5 maintain speed and time increase. Check the weights levels again.	16 April 12 minutes Increased on one machine from 10 kg to 12 kg It's getting easier and on

	4. Repeat points 4 from past two weeks	three occasions I was home before the bus as it was stuck in traffic!
WEEK FOUR	1 Session 6 increase speed by 0.5 2. Session 7 increase time by 2 minutes 3. Increase one weight machine by one level 4. As for last week and go for walk in the park on Sunday	23 April 5.0 mph 15 minutes – need more time to get used to this Maintained weights and feel ready to increase leg machine by one level YESSSSSS!

RESULTS SO FAR AND CELEBRATION

Weights improved on 2 machines
Speed increased
Time on treadmill increased
Speed increased
Have beaten bus home on lots of occasions. Enjoyed walk in the park and we had lunch out at the end.
Ready to push on. Need to ask Graham to check my progress.

It seems easy, doesn't it, but that's because the steps are small. It's a lifestyle change which will hopefully last most of your life, so it's worth taking time to get it right. Yet there may still be reluctance to make that first step. Why is that? We need to explore this in greater depth because this could point a way to what stops you. First ask yourself the following question, *What's stopping me from taking and making that first step?* Is your answer like any of the following:

- not knowing what to do
- not knowing where to start
- not knowing how to do something
- not believing you are capable or will ever be capable
- fear of failure
- fear of success
- unwillingness to enter this new uncharted territory
- excuses: there's not enough time/energy/opportunity/it won't work, it hasn't before
- what's the point?

All of these will sabotage most people's chances of success. But there are ways round these. We've drawn up some ideas:

REASON	IDEAS
Not knowing what to do	Research Ask someone, a friend, a mentor, someone who has already made the changes you want Check out blogs and self-help sites on the internet

	Get creative – write down one hundred things you could do and notice what interests you most
Not knowing where to start	Get imaginative – write down twenty things you could do today from the silly to the serous Ask someone Research Ask yourself 'What is the single most simple thing I could do today that would start to make a difference?' and do it Go to chapter six on *Managing Obstacles* and pick out some ideas
Not knowing how to do something	Research the internet Go on a course Buy a book Ask someone who is an expert or who has already achieved what you want and ask them if they would mind sparing you ten minutes to tell you how they did what they did. For more information on this,

	go to chapter six on *Managing Obstacles* and check out the section called *Modelling: who else knows how to do what you want to do*
Not believing you're capable or will ever be capable	Go to chapter six on *Managing Obstacles*
Fear of failure	See above
Fear of success	See above And explore what it is that's frightening you. Make a list of anything that comes to mind. Something will surprise you and that is what you can take to chapter six *Managing Obstacles*
Excuses; There's not enough time/ energy/ opportunity/it won't work, it hasn't before	Time; take one day and audit how you have spent your time. Where are there examples of lost minutes? How much TV do you honestly watch?

	For any other excuses, refer to the section on *self-talk* in chapter seven
Unwillingness to enter this new uncharted territory	See fear of success
What's the point?	If you are at this stage, we'd suggest you get some help from a counsellor, a trusted and wise colleague, a doctor as this could be a sign of depression and that needs specialist help

We hope that by this time you have a clearer idea of what you plan to do and how it can be achieved but you may still have reservations or have discovered some obstacles. The next chapter, called *Managing Obstacles* provides more ideas.

Chapter six: Managing obstacles

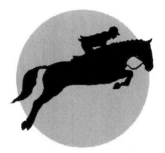

Public Domain Pictures[iv]

You've got your action plan, you've made a start and... something derails you. It can be a variety of other things from life (unexpected change of job, a move, a new relationship, family issues). For some people, these may prove a catalyst for greater action. For others, it may be time to rein back and let the poor old brain focus on the immediate issues. It quickly gets overloaded.

Common reasons for not achieving our goals include:

- goals not being specific enough
- doubts about whether the goal is achievable; and whether success is really deserved

- procrastination – fear of what the future might be like if success happened
- lack of motivation or commitment

The previous chapter, though, *Taking Actions*, has given you tips and techniques for making your goals strong, well founded and motivating.

However, it's possible that other challenges may remain. Did your answer to the question *What's stopping you?* include any of the following responses:

- not believing you're capable or will ever be capable
- fear of failure
- fear of success

If you recognise any of these, it may be that you have a limiting belief. We are not using the word belief in a religious or faith linked. We all have beliefs about the world in which we live, other people, our competencies and our frailties. These beliefs can be useful, such as a belief that other people can be supportive. They can, however, sometimes be less than empowering. Such beliefs are sometimes described as *limiting beliefs* as they can hold you back and limit your potential. We are sure that you could write down a list and it may include some of these which are common.

Examples of limiting beliefs:

- I can't...
- I'm afraid to...

- I'm useless at....
- I'll never...
- I'm hopeless at...
- Someone like me can't...
- I don't deserve...
- I am not (fit/pretty/strong/sexy/rich/popular etc. etc.) enough.

If you want to explore these more and where they might come from, a simple internet search will provide plenty of blogs and websites which will provide this information.

So what can we do about them?

First of all, unless we can recognise and acknowledge them, nothing will happen. It's worthwhile taking some time over this and give yourself some treats too as we could be dealing with possible painful thoughts. Reassure yourself that once you've spotted your limiting belief, you can begin work and sometimes simply recognising them, writing them down and acknowledging them can help. The first thing is once you have identified a limiting belief, write it down. Then try these questions:

What's your outcome?	I want to get fit
What's stopping you?	I've got no willpower

What evidence have you got of your lack of will power? When have you shown will power? Where did you get this belief? Who helped reinforce this belief? What might be a more useful belief? What would you like to believe?	

Most people will be able to flip the language from a limiting belief to an empowering belief such as *I've got no will power* to *I want more willpower*. Making it happen is something else. However, once we've got to this stage, we can start to shift these beliefs.

How to shift limiting beliefs

Some of the following have worked for us. You may find other ideas on the internet or from people you know. The important thing is to have a go and if one thing doesn't work, try another. When we studied NLP (Neuro Linguistic Programming) we learnt that there are three main components to NLP:

- setting outcomes
- acuity to notice if you are getting your outcome
- flexibility to do something else

One of the underlying presuppositions of NLP is that if what you are doing isn't working, do something different. We rather like the quote from Anthony Robbins:

> *If you always do what you've always done, you'll always get what you've always got*

At this point, be prepared to take time and try a lot of things; a lapse of any type is just that – not a collapse and certainly not a relapse. Here are 3 strategies to shift a belief:

1   Sometimes simply writing down the limiting belief can shift it. It may seem ridiculous written in black or blue and white.

2   Using language to shift a belief is a bit like using affirmations. Try this, as the jump from a limiting belief to an empowering belief can sometimes be too large for the brain to deal with. We've included an example:

LIMITING BELIEF	OPPOSITE EMPOWER-ING BELIEF	ADD AN INTEREST WORD	ADD A PROCESS WORD	NEW EMPOWER-ING BELIEF
I'm useless at job interviews	I'm great at interviews	I'm interested/ curious/ intrigued/	I'm interested/ curious/ intrigued/ to discover/ learn/ understand/	I'm interested in learning how to be good at job interviews

			good at interviews	

Is that a better place to start? It gives you the chance to use this as an affirmation or to use as a starting place to discover how you can be better at job interviews.

3. Think about the structure of your belief. What does it feel like when you say it out loud? For this technique, we're indebted to our NLP training and trainers of the past. Simply compare how it feels inside yourself when you say your limiting belief; compared to how it feels inside yourself when you say a positive belief that you know is true.

STATE YOUR LIMITING BELIEF	STATE YOUR EMPOWERING BELIEF
I'm useless at job interviews	I'm great at cooking curry
What does it feel like? Scared Wobbly inside Shaky legs Clammy hands Sick	What does it feel like? Rubbing my hands together Excitement Fingers itch to get chopping and grinding
What do you see?	What do you see?

A big table with lots of people sitting behind it with piles of paper and pens in their hands Dull grey suits A chair on its own	A pile of brightly coloured vegetables A clean work surface Frying pan and knife Lots of jars of spices
What do you hear? My feet tapping over the floor The scrape of a chair Oh damn. I don't want to be here.	What do you hear? The tap tap of cutting and dicing The sizzle of spices Hope this turns out okay

Which one is different? We reckon the internal dialogue is something you could shift. How would it be if instead of thinking *Oh damn. I don't want to be here,* you changed this to *Hope this turns out okay?*

Imagine it and next time, give this a go.

We've mentioned asking an expert for ideas on how they are successful, particularly if they have a skill you wish to adopt or develop. This is more than a casual chat. What we need to find out is what are the key elements in what they do that we don't, those essential tips that will make the difference. Again, we are indebted to the authors and trainers of NLP for the concept of modelling i.e. finding out what that person does, how and perhaps even why because the argument is that if someone else can do it, so can you, within reasonable boundaries of health, fitness, ability and aptitude. There are many examples of modelling using the full NLP method on the internet. Here we give you a simplified version so that you can find out more if you are interested or skip the section and move on.

Modelling: who else already knows how to do what you want to do?

For modelling to work effectively, we need to find a willing exemplar of the skill we wish to adopt. By willing, we mean someone who would be happy to give you half an hour of their valuable time to answer a few questions. These are the sort of questions that you need to ask:

- what are they doing?
- how are they doing it?
- how do they tell if they are being successful?
- what happens if they find themselves not achieving the result they wanted?
- what do they think as they are doing the skill?

Then it's important that you go through the same process with yourselves. We're sure you will find one difference that you can take on board. For example, one person who was very good at managing their budget thought of themselves as their own bank manager and sat down each Sunday with their laptop and checked their expenditure that week. If it was over their expectations, they set a smaller limit. Another person who was good at time management at work used to open an email and deal with it there and then, rather than say *I'll do that later* and when they had a really important piece of work, they cleared their desk so that there were no distractions. Sometimes simple insights like that can work for other people too, including yourself.

By now we hope you have plenty of ideas for achieving your outcomes but there is one other technique we learnt from NLP which we always found useful. It's called the New Behaviour Generator but is sometimes more commonly known as Mental Rehearsal.

Imagine you've decided to go to the gym, but the thought of walking in through the door and signing up gives you the jitters. First write down some alternative course of action;

- email first so they are expecting you
- phone first so they are expecting you
- go to a gym that's further away but where you know some of your work colleagues attend
- ask a friend to workout with you
- tell yourself to do it

After you've written these down, read through each in turn and check out which one feels right. We're asking you to use your sense of feeling here. We all have it... that sinking feeling when you are approaching something you don't want to do, a hunch about a new way of doing something... notice how many are associated with sensations. We use this part of our being lots of times. How often have you heard of someone who is a pain in the neck? Or ever used a phrase such as sick to the stomach?

Are any of these familiar?

When you select an activity, check if it feels right and only you know what that means to you. It might be a warm feeling in your stomach, a feeling like a pat on the shoulder, an ease of any tension over the shoulders or you might even find yourself nodding or saying *yes* out loud.

That's the action to take. Imagine yourself doing it. What will you see, what will you be thinking, saying, feeling? Imagine it in great detail several times. What you're doing is programming the brain so when you take the action it's easier, as your brain thinks you've done it before. Anyone involved in sports will be familiar with this. You can find out more by searching for mental rehearsal online.

There's one other technique that might be of use as you make changes to your life and patterns of behaviour – anchoring. Again, we're grateful to those involved in NLP for the teaching on this. It's a useful technique for those occasions when you are slightly nervous or need a boost of confidence.

Anchoring

Put simply, anchoring is the ability to recall a positive emotion and to use a stimulus (usually a simple action or word) to help you to recall it. So how does this happen?

1. Recall a powerful example of the positive sensation you wish to use
2. Go deeply into the memory and enjoy the sounds, sights, smells, tastes and sensations
3. Use a trigger word or an action which will from now on be associated with this positive experience

4. Enjoy the moment for a few seconds before you come out and do something else for a few moments (shake your body, wiggle your hips, look out of the window, sing happy birthday)
5. Repeat steps 1 to 4
6. When you've gone through these steps a few times more, try doing the action, saying your trigger word or both. Are those same positive feelings starting to creep through your system? You've got an anchor

If this hasn't worked for you, try something else. If you're sceptical, here are some common anchors which we take for granted every day:

- a feeling of excitement on Christmas Eve (memories anchored from childhood)?
- nervousness when you knock on the boss's door?
- the athlete and the starters pistol
- a red traffic light means stop

Still not convinced? Imagine sucking on a lemon – simply the stimulus of imagining the lemon makes our mouth feel odd.

And there are good reasons for this to work. You may never have heard of Edwin Twitmyer but you will probably have come across the term *knee jerk reaction.* In 1902, he published his research on the subject but identified occasions when instead of a hammer hitting the knee and making the leg jerk, it was enough for his subjects to her the sound of a bell and their knee would respond. Ivan Pavlov's work on the dogs and his bells is more often remembered. What they both used was what is described as a stimulus-response model and is at the very heart of the concept of anchoring.

We hope by now you have a number of techniques to support you as you work through your action plan. Next, in order to ramp up our chances of success, we need to move onto the fourth Tool in our Happiness Toolkit: *how our brains work.*

Chapter seven: How our brains work

So, we're now steadily working through our Happiness Toolkit. We've got to the point where we need to understand more about how our brains work, which is Tool 4. With this knowledge, we'll explore how we can use its amazing potential and avoid its possible downsides, to help us achieve our goals and move towards more happiness.

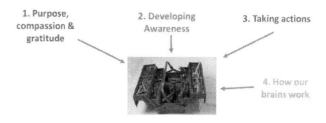

Have you experienced a time when for some curious reason, you found yourself self-sabotaging or doubting that you can achieve certain important things? We want here to focus on self-sabotage and failure because it happens a lot, and there are some very understandable reasons *why* this happens. The answer is that it's all about how our brains are wired, and perhaps sadly, it's just part of being human. So, understanding how our brains are wired is important. Here's an example. For the next minute you're not allowed to think about chocolate – eating it, unwrapping it, popping a square into your mouth and letting it melt on your tongue. And don't forget chocolate biscuits. No, nothing about chocolate must enter your head. Tell yourself, *Don't think about chocolate.*

What's happened? Let's guess. You probably immediately thought about your favourite bar of chocolate! Some of you might even have sneaked off and got a piece? That's fine. You're human and you have a human brain. By finding out more how our brain works, we can learn to handle this sort of situation better and please be reassured, this is all perfectly normal. It's just the way we're all wired.

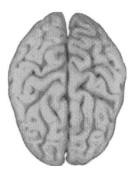

Public Domain Vectors[v]

We carry around a three-pound mass of wrinkly material in our heads that controls every single thing we ever do: from enabling us to think, learn, create, and feel emotions to controlling every blink, breath, and heartbeat – this fantastic control centre is our brain. It's a structure so amazing it was once described as *the most complex thing in the universe* (Murray, 2012). Or as Lyall Watson once said:

> **If the brain were so simple we could understand it, we would be so simple we couldn't**

Our brain is made up of three parts which is why it's referred to as the *Triune Brain* and consists of three interlinked and quite different segments:

- the lizard brain
- the mammal brain
- the human brain

The first brains appeared on the planet about 500 million years ago; and spent a leisurely 430 million years or so evolving into the brains of the earliest primates; and another 70 million years or so evolving into the brains of the first early humans. Then, something happened, suddenly, which resulted in our brains doubling their mass and producing what we now recognize as the human brain. One of the consequences of this pattern of development has left our brains with some built in design faults where there are three distinct, but interconnected parts. These insights come from the pioneering work of neuroscientist Paul McLean (1990), and it was he who first coined the expression *Triune Brain.*

Triune Brain Theory

Lizard Brain	Mammal Brain	Human Brain
Brain stem & cerebelum	Limbic System	Neocortex
Fight or flight	Emotions, memories, habits	Language, abstract thought, imagination, consciousness
Autopilot	Decisions	Reasons, rationalizes

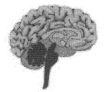 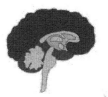

The Triune Brain in Evolution, Paul MacLean, 1960

The lizard brain

The reptilian brain is located deep in our brain stem and is the result of our evolution from life forms of about 500 million years ago, when only reptiles roamed the world. This part of the brain is strongly linked to the spinal cord and is responsible for governing some of the most fundamental functions such as breathing, eating, sleeping, waking up, crying, looking out for and responding to danger, and basic survival. It's in this part of the human brain that the basic instincts of flight or fight are located.

The mammal brain (sometimes called the limbic system)

This part of the brain is unique to mammals. It's existed on the planet for approx. 400 million years. According to MacLean (1990), this part of the brain is the centre of emotion and learning. It developed very early in mammals to regulate the motivations and emotions that we now associate with feeding, reproduction, and attachment behaviours. In MacLean's explanation, the limbic system evaluates everything as either agreeable (pleasure) or disagreeable (pain/distress). Survival is predicated on the avoidance of pain and the repetition of pleasure.

The human brain

This is the youngest part of the brain (approx. 70 million years old). It's also known as the neocortex and it's the one that differentiates us from other animals. It's in charge of planning, anticipating, perceiving time and context, making sense of emotions and giving us the ability to make conscious choices.

Have you ever lost your temper, and afterwards said something to yourself or to others like: *I completely lost it* or *I don't know what came over me?* You are not alone. It's just what we humans do, part of our human experience. The extreme speed of flight or fight behaviours can save our lives if we find ourselves in a dangerous life or death situation, so thank goodness for them. However, as we all know, sometimes the most ancient parts of our brains respond in their lightning fast, strong and automatic ways when they don't need to... For example, when you mislay your car keys and are in a hurry and you wrongly accuse your kids of moving them from their normal place in the house. And then sometimes, we see other people around us who lose it and it's tempting for our own brains to respond in kind, resulting in you suddenly having an argument with someone you love... but for no apparent, logical reason.

So, the key question is: how can we manage these three brains in our heads? First, it helps to know and understand a little bit more about the way the brain works.

- our brain is faster and more powerful than a supercomputer

Your kitten is on the kitchen counter. She's about to step onto a hot stove. You have only seconds to act. Accessing the signals coming from your eyes, your brain quickly calculates when, where, and at what speed you will need to dive to intercept her. Then it orders your muscles to do so. Your timing is perfect and she's safe. No computer can come close to your brain's awesome ability to download, process, and react to the flood of information coming from your eyes, ears, and other sensory organs.

- our brain generates enough electricity to power a lightbulb

Our brain contains about 100 billion microscopic cells called neurons – so many it would take you over 3,000 years to count them all. Whenever you dream, laugh, think, see, or move, it's because tiny chemical and electrical signals are racing between these neurons along billions of tiny neuron highways. Believe it or not, the activity in your brain never stops. Countless messages zip around inside it every second like a supercharged pinball machine. Your neurons create and send more messages than all the phones in the entire world. And while a single neuron generates only a tiny amount of electricity, all your neurons together can generate enough electricity to power a low-wattage bulb.

- neurons send information to our brain at more than 150 miles (241 kilometers) per hour

A bee lands on your bare foot. Sensory neurons in your skin relay this information to your spinal cord and brain at a speed of more than 150 miles (241 kilometres) per hour. Your brain then uses motor neurons to transmit the message back through your spinal cord to your foot to shake the bee off quickly. Motor neurons can relay this information at more than 200 miles (322 kilometres) per hour.

- when we learn, we change the structure of our brain

Riding a bike seems impossible at first. But soon you master it. How? As you practice, your brain sends bike riding messages along certain pathways of neurons over and over, forming new connections. In fact, the structure of your brain changes every time you learn, as well as whenever you have a new thought or memory neurons over and over, forming new connections.

Try this:

Fold your arms. Which arm is on the top? Left or right arm? Now repeat the exercise with the OPPOSITE arm on the top. Does it feel strange? Of course. You're using a different set of skills. Repeat this unfamiliar way of folding your arms a dozen time. Does it feel any different? It may take you a few more repetitions but within a short space of time, this new way is as familiar as the old way. Your brain has learnt.

- exercise helps make us smarter

It's well known that any exercise that makes our heart beat faster, like running or playing basketball, is great for our body and can even help improve our mood. But scientists have recently learned that for a period of time after we've exercised, our body produces a chemical that makes our brain more receptive to learning. So if we're stuck on a tricky problem, going out for walk or just running upstairs before trying the problem again can lead to a solution.

- the power of the unconscious mind

Of all the activity that goes on in our brains, we're only conscious of about ten percent of it. This is called the conscious mind. The other ninety percent of brain activity occurs below the surface of conscious awareness: in our unconscious mind. It's this part of the brain that drives our habits. For example, when we have sometimes driven to work, parked up and then paused to reflect on how we got there, it's our unconscious mind which has done it all for us through sheer force of habit. Imagine how difficult and time consuming it would be if every time we came across a door handle, we had to work out how to open it.

My conscious and my unconscious mind

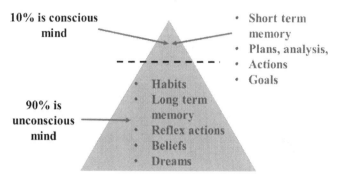

So much of what we do, though, is driven not by conscious thought, but by the *force of habit*, i.e. by unconscious thought. For example, when we stand up and walk, for most of us at least, we just do it without having to think. (Compare that with the image of a toddler who is walking for the first time). Of course, it's useful that our brains have the capacity to automate so much of what we do in life – thus freeing up our brain bandwidth for new ideas and behaviours. Another way of understanding this is to appreciate how easy it is for us to create habits and for large chunks of our lives to be driven by the force of habit.

But here comes the rub, of course. It's as easy to create unhelpful habits as it is to create helpful habits. In fact, given the welter of unending advertising that each person experiences each day, and their focus on things that are often not good for our health and long-term wellbeing, it's probably easier for us to create more unhelpful habits than helpful habits. It follows that a key aspect to being happy with good levels of health and wellbeing is to know how to harness the brain's ability to create habits that serve us well. How do we do this? First, we need to create positive habits.

Creating positive habits

We all know the power that habits can have in our lives and the lives of others. If we have ever commuted to work on the train, we may have spotted how so many of us tend to want to sit in the same compartment or how, given a choice of type of coffee drink, most of us tend to opt for our favourite.

One of the most influential doctors and writers on personal health is Dr Rangan Chatterji, who, in addition to being a practising GP, has worked as the BBC Breakfast health expert. In his book *Feel Better in 5: Your Daily Plan to Feel Great for Life,* Dr Chatterji refers to research that shows that at least fifty percent of all that we all do is driven by habits. As he says:

We are our habits

Another inspirational phrase he sometimes uses is:

Your lifestyle can be your medicine

He goes on to say that the key to health and wellbeing is to take tiny positive steps, each day; and that the ripple effect of these can have a significant effect on our general health and well-being. He suggests that we each take five minutes, three times a day, five days per week, to take small actions which are good for our mind, our body and our heart.

Dr Chatterji offers six top tips to help people to establish such new habits:

- start easy
- connect each health snack to an existing habit
- respect your own rhythm
- design your environment
- use positive self talk
- celebrate your success

He suggests that we each take three (x five minutes) snacks a day:

- a mind health snack
- a body health snack
- a heart health snack

Examples would be:

Example of a Mind Health Snack	Reflecting on yesterday, what you achieved and what you learnt
Example of a Body Health Snack	Two sets of press ups or physical stretches
Example of a Heart Health Snack	Reflecting on your blessings and what you're grateful for

Habits are driven by our unconscious minds: and a key part of personal happiness is to harness its fantastic power. And a good way to do is through making tiny but repeated positive habits in the way suggested by Dr Chatterji.

Another well known and highly respected thinker on self development is Stephen Covey, who emphasises the role of using the positive power of good habits, in his best selling book *The Seven Habits of Highly Effective People.* Covey's work focusses not on eliminating bad habits but on building up good ones. Changing our habits can change not only the way we see the world, but the way the world sees us. His work has lasted the test of time and has helped millions of people. The seven habits are:

1: Be proactive
2: Begin with the end in mind
3: Put first things first
4: Think win/win
5: Seek first to understand, then to be understood
6: Synergize
7: Sharpen the saw

Dr Covey has a useful website which contains lots of helpful tips at:

https://www.franklincovey.com

And next up, is another habit (good or bad) which plays a big part in our personal happiness in life: sleep. It's surely one of the most underestimated and under appreciated tonics for our mind and body and is totally free and available to everyone on a daily basis. Yet so often, it's overlooked.

Importance of Sleep

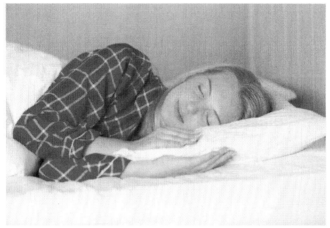

Public Domain Pictures[vi]

We spend (or should spend) about a third of our lives asleep. Sleep is essential – it's as important to our bodies as eating, drinking and breathing, and is vital for maintaining good mental and physical health. Sleeping helps us to recover from mental as well as physical exertion.

Sleep and health are strongly related – poor sleep can increase the risk of having poor health, and poor health can make it harder to sleep. Sleep disturbances can be one of the first signs of distress. Common mental health problems like anxiety and depression can often underpin sleep problems.

The Sleep Foundation (www.sleep foundation.org) make a clear link between the immune system and the quality of our sleep. They say that whilst more sleep won't necessarily prevent us from getting sick, skimping on it could adversely affect our immune system, leaving us susceptible to a bad cold, a case of the flu – or even worse Without sufficient sleep, our bodies make fewer proteins known as cytokines. This is a type of protein that targets infection and inflammation, effectively creating an immune response. Cytokines are both produced and released during sleep, causing a double whammy if you skimp on sleep. Chronic sleep loss even makes the flu vaccine less effective by reducing our body's ability to respond.

We all know about the myth of telling people to get out of bed and pull themselves together, but lethargy, tiredness, and disturbed sleep can be part of having a mental health problem or a side effect of taking medication. Addressing sleep and sleep disorders as part of mental health treatment is very important and can be overlooked.

One of the most influential researchers on sleep was Dr William Dement, formerly of the Sleep Research Center at Stanford University. He was one of the world's leading scientists on sleep and was part of the team in the 1950s who discovered REM (Rapid Eyeball Movement) and its link to dreaming. An updated version of his original website which contains lots of useful material on sleep is:

www.End-Your-Sleep-Deprivation.com

Dr Dement introduced the concept of the triangle of health:

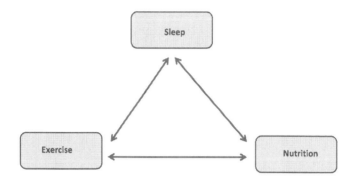

The triangle of health, (or triumvirate, as he refers to it), calls for eating well, exercising enough, and sleeping right. He says that people tend to have a great understanding of the importance of exercise and nutrition, but healthy sleep knowledge and good practice is too often lacking. The connections between these three elements provide the ultimate basis for well-being and happiness. A person who behaves according to its three principles – good nutrition, physical fitness, and healthy sleep – is well on their way to optimized health, energy, and longevity.

Also, a lot goes on whilst we are asleep. In a typical night's sleep we have significant changes in brain wave activity – recurring cycles each lasting approx. ninety minutes each, during which time our brain activity changes from "normal" to very slow:

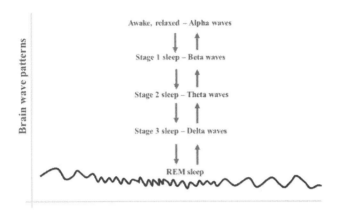

When the brain is in deep sleep, the brain waves are very slow (0.5 – 3 Hz), during which time our eyeballs move quite fast (flutter) and when we dream. This kind of sleep pattern (REM pattern) happens ninety minutes after we fall asleep. The first period of REM typically lasts ten minutes. Each of our later REM stages gets longer, and the final one may last up to an hour. Our heart rate and breathing quickens.

We need approx. four REM cycles each night. Add about thirty minutes of getting into sleep, and thirty minutes waking up, we're roughly at seven hours, which is close to the amount of sleep the average adult needs per night.

Babies can spend up to fifty percent of their sleep in the REM stage, compared to only about twenty percent for adults. According to the National Sleep Foundation, newborns spend about fifty percent out of their twelve to sixteen hour sleep time in the REM stage. We know that new neural connections are formed in the REM stage, and this may be the reason why babies need it so much.

There are numerous studies (one of which is from Matthew Walker, 2017) suggesting the benefits of those who get enough REM sleep:

- We're better able to read other people's emotions:
  It's been proven that after reaching REM sleep, people are more able to recognize emotions on photographs showing various facial expressions.

- Our emotional response to stress is lower:
  It seems that after a good night's rest our emotional centre in the brain is less sensitive and more able to cope with difficult situations.

- There's a lower risk of developing Alzheimer's disease:
  During sleep, our brain clears out certain neurotoxins, including those found in Alzheimer's disease patients. Having plenty of sleep may be connected with lowering the risk of this disease.

- It may improve memory:
  A study has shown that REM sleep deprivation in rats reduces proliferation of cells in the part of the brain which takes part in long-term memory.

- It helps learning and cognition:
  Getting the needed REM sleep is linked to better learning – individuals who were not able to reach REM demonstrated an inability to reproduce what they had been taught before falling asleep.

- It improves our mood:
  Not only does REM make us less prone to stress, but it also replenishes neurotransmitters that are responsible for good mood – serotonin and dopamine.

- It may enhance creativity:
  Some studies have shown that problem solving capability was higher in those who have had REM sleep.

When we don't get enough sleep one night, we accumulate what's known as a *sleep debt*. If the trend of not achieving our daily sleep requirement continues, our sleep debt continues to increase accordingly, further degrading our performance throughout the day.

We can think of sleep debt like a growing weight over us that we have to carry around throughout the day. Unless paid back, the debt gets bigger and bigger while we're awake until... *Suddenly!!! We're asleep!*

In order to feel fully rested again, and to achieve *optimal alertness* throughout the day, there's one long-term solution that never fails: we must repay our sleep debt hour for hour. To re-emphasize what was mentioned above, our sleep debt will continue to accumulate over days, weeks, and months without diminishing, unless we do something about it. This is sometimes easier said than done, but the importance of doing so is paramount. Far and away the most important aspect of the regulation of sleep is the following simple fact: *sleep loss is cumulative.* When total nightly sleep is reduced by exactly the same amount each night for several consecutive nights, the tendency to fall asleep in the daytime becomes progressively stronger each day, and performance is often compromised as a result.

Sleep debt:

- Decreases our alertness and ability to maintain focus:
  Carrying a sizable sleep debt throughout the day can drastically decrease productivity. Fatigue will compromise your attention, and as a result cognitive performance will suffer. Specifically, learning, memory, and creativity are frequently hampered by a large sleep debt. In a situation such as driving a car this decreased alertness can, and has repeatedly, led to fatal results.
- Destabilises our mood:
  It's not uncommon for sleep-deprived individuals to be subject to extreme emotions and mood swings. A very tired person who is laughing uncontrollably at one moment may be crying or yelling angrily a few minutes later.
- Decreases our energy and motivation:
  A decrease in energy and motivation is probably the most noticeable consequence of sleep deprivation. Individuals who have not received sufficient sleep will feel lethargic and uninspired to work.

- Reduces control and coordination but increases impulsiveness:
  A lack of sleep is often associated with changes in bodily control. Tired individuals often feel enhanced physical impulses, such as an otherwise inexplicable desire to eat.
- Can cause us pain:
  Extreme sleep deprivation can literally cause a degree of physical pain, such as headaches.

With the tendency for a lot of people to be attached to their mobile phones, tablets and other devices, as well as the TV, there's now research (by Monique LeBourgeois in the journal *Pediatrics,* November 2017) which shows the effect this is having on their sleep habits, and overall well-being. This research found adverse associations between screen time and sleep health – primarily because of later bedtimes and less time spent sleeping, psychological stimulation from content consumed and the negative impact of screen light on sleep patterns.

The NHS has some helpful recommendations to promote effective sleep habits. They are:

Sleep at regular times

This programmes the brain and internal body clock to get used to a set routine. Most adults need between six and nine hours of sleep every night. By working out what time you need to wake up, you can set a regular bedtime schedule. It's also important to wake up at the same time every day. While it may seem like a good idea to try to catch up on sleep after a bad night, doing so on a regular basis can also disrupt your sleep routine.

<u>Make sure you wind down</u>

Winding down is a critical stage in preparing for bed. There are lots of ways to relax:

- taking a warm bath (not hot) will help your body reach a temperature that's ideal for rest
- writing *to do* lists for the next day can organise your thoughts and clear your mind of any distractions
- doing relaxation exercises, such as light stretching that you might do in yoga, help to relax the muscles. (Vigorous exercise, however, will have the opposite effect.)
- listening to relaxation scripts or gentle hypnotic music and sound effects
- reading a book or listening to the radio relaxes the mind by distracting it
- avoiding using smartphones, tablets or other electronic devices for an hour or so before you go to bed as the light from the screen on these devices may have a negative effect on sleep.

If you'd like a bit more detail about how your sleep habits can shape up, there's a free online quiz.

https://psychcentral.com/quizzes/sleep-quiz/

Finally, what do we conclude from all this? The brutal truth is that without good quality and quantity sleep habits, our chances of living a happy and fulfilled life are low, if not impossible.

How many times have you found yourself lying awake at night, tossing and turning in bed? What's the one thing we can guarantee that's happening, as we lie there in bed? Our self-talk will be going round in our heads, constantly....

That's what we turn to next.

Self-talk

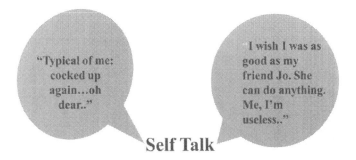

"Typical of me: cocked up again...oh dear.."

I wish I was as good as my friend Jo. She can do anything. Me, I'm useless.."

Self Talk

Most of us are in constant mental chatter. We talk to ourselves all day long and, unfortunately, this self-talk is frequently negative. Often, it's tainted with guilt about our past or anxiety about our future. This negativity can destroy any seed of hope that we may otherwise have in striving for our dreams. Our actions are inspired by our thoughts. If we can change the way we think, we can begin to change the actions we take. Practicing positive self-talk can help us set in motion actions that will bring us greater rewards.

The following are three steps to positive self-talk. By following these steps you'll begin to rid your inner conversations of negativity and instead have empowering thoughts. This should make it easier for you to achieve your goals. After all, no one wants to set out on changes and be bombarded with thoughts such as *You'll fail. You'll never do this. It's too hard.* We're sure you can insert many more from your own experience. The first step in dealing with this negative self-talk is to become aware of it.

- eliminate internal negative chatter

A common negative talk involves saying *I can't.* When we say this or *it's too difficult*, we are creating a resistance. Having such a mental block will prevent us from achieving a task we could otherwise succeed at. Anytime we catch ourselves saying *I can't...* we need to turn around and challenge this claim with, *Why can't I?* But it'll not be easy to make a switch if we have a long history or negative self-talk. Our self-talk has probably become negative over the years due to various factors. For instance, if our first teacher repeatedly told us we were stupid, it will be hard not to believe them. Our inner chatter will be filled with talk of *I'm so slow* and *It's so hard to learn.* If we voice such negative stories, our actions are going to result in low self-esteem.

- positive affirmations

Affirmations are positive statements of a desired outcome or goal. They are usually short, believable and focused. By repeating them over and over again, we build inroads into our unconscious mind, opening up the possibility of a new state of thoughts. An important step when repeating affirmations is to read the affirmations aloud with feeling. The mere reading of the words bears no consequence unless we put some emotions behind them. Why? Our unconscious mind takes any orders given in complete faith. So, the daily practice of repeating affirmations is important. Initially we may be sceptical toward the statement of the positive affirmation. However, if we follow this simple set of instructions, scepticism will soon give way to a new set of beliefs and then crystallized into absolute faith.

- positive scripts

And here's another thing about negative self-talk. It can, over time, spin a drama that traps and limits us in life. Here's an alternative. Create an uplifting story that runs like a movie script. Some visualization will be helpful. Build on a story with a positive outline. The longer we can tell this story to our self, the better. It is also best if we can make this story about having our goals achieved. When we do this, we start to internalize our goals and dreams, as if they are something already achieved. We explore more in **chapter ten** the concept of life scripts.

These mysterious and wonderful workings of the brain have been fascinating neuroscientists, researchers and writers a lot in the last twenty years or so, resulting in a number of useful new ideas about how the brain works and how to get the best out of it. One such writer is Dr Steve Peters, a consultant psychiatrist who coached some of the British Olympic Cycling

Team, (such as Chris Hoy and Victoria Pendleton). In 2012, he wrote a book called The Chimp Paradox.

The Chimp Paradox

In his book *The Chimp Paradox,* Steve Peers draws attention to the Triune Brain (see chapter seven); and compared the lizard and mammal brain's ultra-quick, ultra-strong and ultra-alarmist responses to any perceived threats or dangers to the behaviour of a *chimp.*

Steve Peters goes on to explain that the ancient parts of the brain (the lizard and mammal parts which have evolved over millennia) are designed to process information with feelings and impressions; and then go on to use emotional thinking to respond to events, especially those they interpret (rightly or wrongly) as threats. And the brain does this at huge speed, often resulting in us feeling suddenly overwhelmed with negative emotion such as fear, anger or panic. It's these parts of the brain that he calls the *chimp* brain.

On the other hand, there is a more recently evolved part of our brain, which is run by logic and which Peters calls the *human* part of the brain. Our job as well-adjusted humans, Peters says, is to use our logical *human* brain to understand what's going on in our *chimp* brain and to appreciate and value what it is doing for us, which is seeking to protect us from potential danger. It's as if we have two brains in there, each with their own distinct style of thinking, as the diagram below shows:

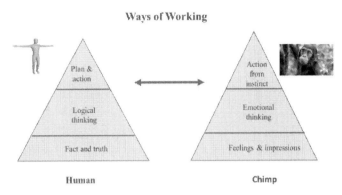

Ways of Working

Human — Plan & action / Logical thinking / Fact and truth

Chimp — Action from instinct / Emotional thinking / Feelings & impressions

From Steve Peters *Chimp Paradox*

Steve Peters leaves us with this sobering thought:

> *Managing our impulsive, emotional chimp as an adult will be one of the biggest factors determining how successful we are in life*

The metaphor of the *chimp* is a powerful and useful tool. In addition to his book, Steve Peters has posted several YouTube clips on his approach which are easy to find with a simple search. Put together with all the other insights, tools and techniques in this book, Steve Peters' insights and his *chimp* model can go a long way towards helping us to understand ourselves and others better, and thus producing more success and happiness.

So why does this all this unhelpful activity occur in the brain? Surely, we control our thoughts, don't we?

The SCARF model

Another leading neuroscientist in this area is David Rock, the author of *Your Brain at Work*. David is the Director of the Neuroleadership Institute and has identified the brain's need for Status, Certainty, Autonomy, Relatedness and Fairness (SCARF).

We have already seen how that little thing we call the brain which nestles in our heads has evolved over hundreds of millions of years from the early days of the reptiles. Over this time, it has perhaps not surprisingly developed some very strong patterns and instincts, one of which, David Rock reminds us, is how our brain's natural instinct is to classify the world around us into things that may (a) hurt us, or (b) help us to stay alive. To minimise danger and maximise reward. And so the brain constantly scans the world, telling us what to pay attention to, generating emotions such as fear, danger, anxiety, curiosity, pleasure and joy. But overall, the strongest emotions which the brain tends to generate most and first of all are those which are designed to keep us safe, i.e. fear and anxiety.

We are the descendants of people who paid lots of attention when there was even a tiny rustle in the woods – in a dangerous world, only the most vigilant survived. Over the millennia, the brain has learnt to excel at spotting danger, and reacts amazingly quickly if it spots danger. Human beings *walk* towards, but *run* away.

So if you are having difficulties with achieving your outcomes, are they all posed in the positive? Are they in the negative or both? It may be that you are one of the people who need to know the positive and negative outcomes of your changed actions. For example, if you want to get fitter, could it be that your outcome is *to be able to play with the grandkids?* That's fine. If you're struggling, what might the effect be if you include an *away from* motivation so your outcome is *to be able to play with the grandkids and not get worn out after five minutes*?

David Rock's research has gone on to identify five specific factors that the human brain is designed to run away from, or walk towards, and these are:

- how we perceive our status
- the degree of certainty or uncertainty we experience in any situation
- the amount of autonomy we experience in any situation
- the degree to which we feel connected to, or disconnected from, others
- the fairness or unfairness we perceive in any situation

This model has since come to be called SCARF, and is a very useful shorthand for what the brain tends to spot in any situation, with the resulting release of emotions which then flood into our bodies and can sabotage any chances of successful change.

SCARF Model of Social Threats and Rewards

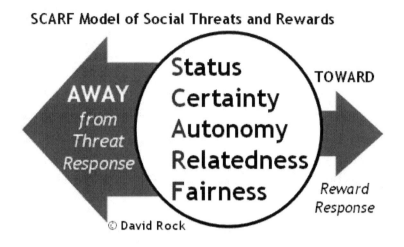

Have you ever felt *left out* or excluded from a group or family activity? When this kind of thing happens, we all know how it can make us feel… upset, hurt or angry. This is an example of the SCARF model coming into play. When we feel like this, it hurts because our brain spots a threat to our status and relatedness. Research has shown that this response can stimulate the same region of the brain as physical pain. In other words, our brain is sending out the signal that we're in danger. Furthermore, when we feel threatened – either physically or socially – the release of cortisol (the stress hormone) affects our creativity and productivity. We literally can't think straight, and this increases the feeling of being threatened. On the flip side, when we feel rewarded (for instance, when we receive praise for our work) our brains release dopamine – the happy hormone. Of course, we want more! So we seek out ways to be rewarded again.

We're going to explain these in turn:

Status

These days, we get bombarded by adverts… and of course one of the main aims of adverts is to encourage us all to do what others are doing or to have what the adverts tell us others have got. In other words, a lot of adverts play on the brain's natural instinct to spot dangers to our well-being: the *Fear of Missing Out* (FOMO). It used to be called *Keeping up with the Joneses* i.e. maintaining and increasing our status.

Another example where the brain may spot a threat to our status is if we think we are on the wrong end of some feedback. Sadly, this happens a lot in the workplace. And when this happens, it can leave us feeling deeply wounded. It may even cause us to become angry and defensive. A gentler approach could help here. For instance, we could offer the person the chance to evaluate their own performance first or try to reframe any feedback in a more positive way.

The other side of the coin is that the brain is also designed to spot positive examples of where you feel your status is increased. So, for example, at work or in families, the more you give genuine, positive praise when they perform well, and provide them with opportunities to develop their skills and knowledge, the brain releases the 'happy chemical' dopamine, which then encourages more of the same positive behaviours.

Certainty

Even though the natural state of the world is for things to change and time to move on, most of us often crave for more stability and certainty. Most of us have experienced time at work when there seems to be constant re-organisation, and with it, lots of uncertainty. The reason most of want more stability and certainty is that our 'ancient' brain sees change as a threat, possibly to our survival. When we're uncertain of something, the frontal cortex of our brains starts to work overtime as it attempts to make sense of the unknown. This can cause us to feel threatened and to lose focus, releasing the stress hormone chemicals. As you are embarking on some major life changes, you will be experiencing this uncertainty. Will it work? What will happen if it does. Or doesn't?

The human brain prefers predictability. When we know what to expect, we feel safe. This safety is a reward in itself, and at work or in families, we can maximize it by being clear on what we expect from each team or family member. This will give them direction, and they'll feel safe in the knowledge that they're on the right track, no matter how uncertain the wider environment is.

Autonomy

Most of us know how it feels to be micromanaged: possibly resentful, hurt and grumpy. The ancient brain automatically seeks an environment where you have enough scope to take action under your own steam, rather than under the rule of someone else. If the brain spots any examples of micromanagement, where you may be over controlled by others, it will generate the Threat Response, releasing into the body the classic stress hormones. Issues of control v autonomy provide a classic dilemma for most parents, i.e. how much freedom do you give to your children versus how much control? On the other hand, the brain does respond well to times when it feels it is being trusted to take autonomous action, and to use initiative, releasing the happy chemical dopamine. This is why it was important to identify changes that are within your locus of control. (Refer back to chapter four).

Relatedness

In theory, we live in an interconnected world, with extensive use of the internet, Wi-Fi, and mobile phones, and yet in the UK, loneliness is a major issue for lots of people. Research by Holt-Lunstad 2010 shows that loneliness, living alone and poor social connections are as bad for our health as smoking twenty-five cigarettes a day, and that loneliness is worse for us than obesity. Data from Age UK shows us that the number of over fifties experiencing loneliness is set to reach 2 million by 2015/26. Younger adults aged sixteen to twenty-four years report feeling lonely more often than those in older age groups. Women often report feeling lonely more often than men. Those single or widowed are at particular risk of experiencing loneliness more often. **The ancient brain is designed to see safety in numbers, with the tribe, fully connected.** If the brain spots a lack of relatedness, it can leave us feeling isolated and unhappy. This can reduce creativity, commitment and collaboration. On the other hand, the brain is good at spotting when we connect well with others, releasing the hormone oxytocin (also known as the 'love hormone'). The more oxytocin that's released, the more connected we feel.

Fairness

How often have we witnessed a toddler in anger and frustration, stamping their feet and exclaiming: "It's not fair!!". Again, this gives us a good illustration of how even the toddler brain is excellent at spotting examples of perceived unfairness and flooding the body with the stress hormones that create the feelings of anger and frustration. If someone believes something to be unfair, it will activate their neocortex – the region of the brain that is linked to disgust. This results in a powerful threat response. On the other hand, the brain does respond well to situations where fairness prevails. So, in families or at work, the brain likes it when individual goals and roles, hierarchy, and day-to-day operations, can remedy this.

Finally, we end this chapter with a reminder of how our brains are so very intimately connected up with our feelings and bodies.

The Mind/Body Connection

The human body is a great example of how different parts interact with each other, not least when we think about the mind, our feelings and our body. Each organ in our body, such as our heart and our lungs, function on their own, but also in deep connection with all the other organs inside us. This means, for example, that we can change the way we feel by changing what we think, and what's happening in our bodies affects our thoughts and feelings.

Mind and Body Connection

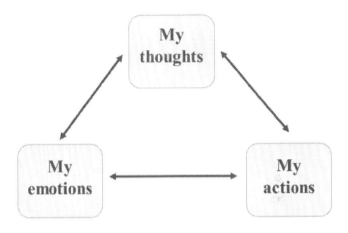

So, if we think about an important presentation or interview that we have to do, this can create significant changes in the hormones inside us, which in turn can change our feelings. If we do something kind for someone else, like going shopping for them, it can change our internal chemistry which in turn can create positive emotions and thoughts in our heads.

We all know what it's like to imagine something like sucking on a lemon! This simple act of imagination can make our mouths feel funny, i.e. can change our behaviour and our internal feelings. Equally, if we imagine eating our favourite food, we can find ourselves salivating, and feeling better. Of course, there are upsides here and potential downsides. The reason some people drink too much, or take drugs is to change this internal chemistry, which in turn can change any feelings and thoughts about life. On the other hand, we can choose to use this interconnected thinking for good and to create more happiness.

And finally...

Twenty or thirty years ago, we may have often heard the term *hard wired* to describe how the brain works, but much of more recent research on the brain has shown that the brain is very able to develop and grow, just like any other muscle. The term that is often used instead to describe the brain is neuroplasticity, i.e. able to grow and develop new cells and connections, depending on how we use it.

> ***Every man can, if he so desires, become the sculptor of his own brain***
>
> Santiago Ramon y Cajal (1887)

Neuroplasticity is the brain's ability to change, remodel and reorganize for the purpose of better ability to adapt to new situations. So, just as many of us are keen to get fit physically, and build muscle where it's needed, so too, we can choose if we wish, to stretch and grow the brain in our heads, not least by taking action to develop ourselves, and build positive habits to increase happiness.

So far, in this book, we have explored four of the Tools in the Happiness Toolkit:

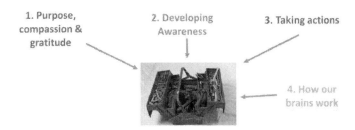

These tools, once applied and embedded into our daily lives, can make a huge difference to our overall happiness. Next, we're going to explore our fifth Tool in the Happiness Toolkit: how we can increase our understanding and skills in how we communicate (with ourselves and others), and in so doing add even more to our success, as well as helping others.

Chapter eight: Enhancing our communication skills

And now, onto our fifth Tool from the Happiness Toolkit: *enhancing our communication skills*.

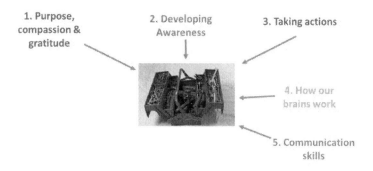

1. Purpose, compassion & gratitude

2. Developing Awareness

3. Taking actions

4. How our brains work

5. Communication skills

The language we use helps us understand and make sense of the world. Sometimes, though, the way we use language can inadvertently create traps, which if we were more aware of what was going on inside our heads, we could avoid. That's what this chapter is all about. It will give us some tools to help use language more effectively, giving us new options in life: because the words we use have *power*:

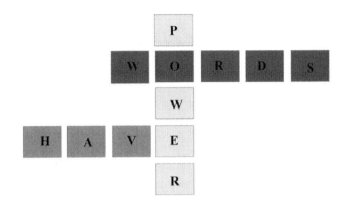

Patterns in the Language We Use

Imagine this scenario:

You meet up with a close friend for a cup of coffee: a person you know is going through a sticky patch in life. After exchanging the usual pleasantries, they start to describe to you the *awful* day they have just had. You know the first thing you must do is to simply listen and show empathy.

Another awful day. Surrounded by idiots at work. My boss did his usual trick of not having time to see me, and then sending me curt emails. He never appreciates anything I do. Usual story, I'm afraid. Nothing in my life is going well at the moment...

Of course, you listen well, but you suspect that your friend may have unconsciously created a somewhat overly pessimistic view of their day. You want to help them and you know that one way to do this, in addition to good quality listening, is to ask some delicate questions which, you hope, might help your friend get a more balanced view of their day – and thus be a bit happier.

You happen to know that your friend has a close and supportive small team who work for them. You decide to focus your friend's attention on this small team, since you suspect there is great work going on here, and by noticing this, your friend will realise that his statement, *surrounded by idiots,* is an over generalisation and distortion.

So, you say to your friend: *Tell me about how your small support team are doing – I seem to recall that in the past, they've done sterling work.*

Your friend's mood instantly lifts as he tells you about the great work his support team did today (and the tenor of the whole conversation improves).

You next decide to hear more about the boss, since clearly your friend's relationship with the boss is important. One word in your friend's opening statement that sticks with you is the word *never* regarding showing appreciation, and your hunch is that your friend may unintentionally be over generalising and deleting some good examples of positive feedback received.

So, you say to your friend: *I'm sorry to hear about your boss – he sounds as if he's having a tough time too. Tell me, are there not specific times in the year when you both sit down, and have a quality feedback conversation?*

Your friend pauses for a moment and then tells you that yes, they do have a formal appraisal system, and yes, your friend and the boss did have a useful feedback conversation only last month, when the boss was most appreciative of your friend and their team's efforts.

Again, your friend's mood lifts, and you both order another nice cup of coffee...

So, what's going on here? In 1975, John Grinder and Richard Bandler researched the way humans use language to make sense of the world and discovered three recurring patterns we all use:

- generalisations
- deletions
- distortions

Often, we use such patterns in a way which helps us in our lives, but sometimes we find ourselves using these patterns in an unhelpful way. Being aware of these patterns, both in our own lives and noticing others use of them can make a significant contribution towards our happiness.

We'll look at each of these patterns in turn:

Generalisations

> *I often wonder why the whole world is so prone to generalise. Generalisations are seldom if ever true and are utterly inaccurate*
>
> Agatha Christie (1930)

Have you ever heard someone (or yourself) say something like:

- *I always screw thing up*
- *You never help me out*
- *People here are always so stupid*

Such statements are generalisations. Our ability to generalise is essential when it comes to making sense of the world. Using previous experiences that are similar as a starting point allows us to learn quickly. Imagine if every time you went to open a new door, you had to stop and figure out exactly how to do it: we just use our past experience to generalise how all doors open and close. Sometimes, though, our minds make generalisations that aren't useful or valid. For example, we've had a bad experience of getting our car serviced, and we then generalise up to conclude that all garages are poor quality. Clearly, not true, and a way of thinking that produces a black and white view of the world.

Whether it's in our own self talk, or in conversations with other people, a useful skill is to spot when a generalisation is being made which may not be serving you or the other person well. In which case, the skill is in (a) spotting the generalisation and in (b) challenging it, to reveal a truer and more useful description of the reality.

Imagine a situation where someone who lacks confidence in themselves says to you: *I've got this job interview tomorrow, but I'm really anxious because I never do well in stressful situations.*

The word *never* is the clue that there's a generalisation in here. And, of course, it might not be one hundred percent true. As their friend, colleague or family member, you might want to help this person challenge the generalisation and uncover some situations in their past when they've succeeded in stressful situations, in order that they realise their strengths more. There are probably several ways of challenging this generalisation, including:

Great news about the job interview! Interesting what you say about never doing well in stressful situations. I'm interested to know how this squares with your success in... [doing the triathlon] etc.

Really... never?

Great news about the job interview. I'm interested to know more about those key moments in your life when you have succeeded against the odds?

Example of generalisation	Examples of the language you might choose to challenge the generalisation
I've got this job interview tomorrow, but I'm really anxious because I never do well in stressful situations.	*Never?* *Tell me more about times when you've succeeded in stressful situations.*

	What about that time when you... [add details] *I'm wondering if you may have overlooked the times when you have actually succeeded well?*

Next, we move onto deletions.

Deletions

> **Our nervous system is being fed with more than 2 million pieces of information every second. To make sense of this, we need to delete most of this; and focus our attention on just a small subset of it**
> B Lewis and F Pucelik (1990)

And so, since at any moment in time there's so much that we could possibly pay attention to: for example, the temperature in the room, the noise of the TV in the corner, the traffic passing by in the road, what other family members are up to, what your partner is saying to you, and what the dog is doing (or about to do)... Thankfully, perhaps, we know the brain is designed to have a strict limit on the number of things it can pay attention to at any moment in time. Research in the 1950s by George Miller revealed that on average, our conscious brain can hold only seven (plus or minus two) things in our heads at any given time. As a result, we are constantly tuning into certain aspects of our experience and filtering out others.

When we think of all the hundreds (or more!) things around us that we could possibly pay attention to at any moment in time, it's not surprising to know that thankfully, our brains filter out lots of the available information and focus instead on a small subset of it.

Whether it's in our own self-talk, or in conversations with other people, a useful skill is to spot when a deletion is being made which may not be serving you or that other person well. As with generalisations, the skill is in (a) spotting the deletion and in (b) challenging it, to reveal a truer and more useful description of the reality.

Imagine a situation where someone says to you: *Peter is the very worst boyfriend.* You spot, through the use of the word *worst,* that the person is making a comparison but has deleted key information about who the boyfriend is being compared to. You suspect that it might help the person to be clear about who the boyfriend is being compared to. And so, as their friend, colleague or family member, you might want to help this person challenge the deletion and reveal the deleted information. In this situation, you might want to ask something like:

Hm, I can see your frustration, but tell me, in saying he's the very worst boyfriend, who exactly are you comparing Peter to right now?

The answer to this question might reveal a number of interesting bits of information, including for example that

Peter is the very first boyfriend this person has had and this, in turn, might help the person to reframe how they think of the situation.

Here's another example. Imagine a situation where someone says to you: *I'm fed up.* You spot that the person is clearly deleting some key information. And so, as their friend, colleague or family member, you might want to help this person challenge the deletion and reveal the deleted information. In this situation, you might want to ask something like:

I'm sorry to hear you're fed up. But I'm wondering exactly what or who you're fed up with?

The answer to this question will reveal some key bits of information, which, when you explore it more with the person concerned, might help them to reframe how they think of the situation.

Example of deletion	Examples of the language you might choose to challenge the deletion
Peter is the very worst boyfriend	*Hm, I can see your frustration, but tell me, in saying he's the very worst boyfriend, who exactly are you comparing Peter to right now?*
I'm fed up	*I'm sorry to hear you're fed up. But I'm wondering exactly what or who you're fed up with?*

He hurt me	*Sorry to hear that. I'm curious to know how exactly he hurt you*
They don't care	*May I please ask you some questions about this. Who exactly doesn't care, and about what specifically? And what's your evidence for this?*

And finally, we look next at distortions.

<u>Distortions</u>

> ***We don't see things as they are: we see them as we are***
> Anais Nin

When we speak, we often need to simplify an experience to make sense of it, which can sometimes lead to unintended distortions. Sometimes we don't have all the information and we jump to conclusions that might not always be justified. This isn't necessarily a bad thing – it can create new ways of seeing things, leading to new discoveries and inventions.

Steve Bull in his book *The Game Plan* has a helpful term for this behaviour: *crooked thinking*. And he traces this term back to the work of Dr Albert Ellis, who in the 1950s made the link between how people's beliefs affect their moods. Steve Bull's 5 types of crooked thinking are set out below:

Crooked Thinking Type (adapted from Dr A Ellis)	Examples of self defeating crooked thinking
Not Fair thinking	*Things really shouldn't be like this. It's not fair. I don't deserve this treatment*
Driver thinking	*I absolutely must perform well tomorrow to avoid a disaster. If I don't, it will be an utter disaster*
Stopper thinking	*I'm useless. I can't do it. I'm going to screw things up*
Illogical thinking	*If this happens, then that will surely follow. If I make a mistake, they will hold it against me for year*

***Blaming* thinking**	*It's his fault. It's her fault. It's everyone's fault. It's not my fault!*

A lot of this crooked thinking occurs in our heads when we talk to ourselves (see chapter seven which deals with self-talk) – it's normal human behaviour. Even the great golfer Nick Faldo, the six times Golf Major winner and Britain's greatest golfer does so. In his own words:

> *My game depends on focus and concentration. While I'm playing, I'm talking to myself inside my head the whole time, issuing verbal commands to myself. Sometimes the conversation comes out, and I'll literally be talking to myself. I'll be saying "Right, come on, get the f*** on with it, concentrate you dick. Go on there, my son, rotate, turn and now…hit*

Nick Faldo quote from <u>www.azquotes.com</u>

Having reviewed the 5 different types of crooked thinking, it's important to consider when and where we might be inclined to slip into such language and thinking. In the table below, there are some examples of self-defeating crooked thinking we might well have said to ourselves, or even heard other people saying to us. And in the right-hand column, we suggest some possible ways to challenge the crooked thinking, either for ourselves or for other people:

Crooked Thinking Type	Examples of self-defeating crooked thinking	Possible ways to challenge this crooked thinking
Not Fair thinking	Things really shouldn't be like this. It's not fair. I don't deserve this treatment	*Tell me: what do you want instead of this; and what specifically are you going to do to change things for the better?*
Driver thinking	I absolutely must perform well tomorrow to avoid a disaster. If I don't, it will be an utter disaster	*Is it possible that you might be exaggerating a bit here? How can you make sure you do the best you can? That's all you can do, you know*
Stopper thinking	I'm useless. I can't do it. I'm going to screw things up	*What's a more useful thing you could say to yourself? Help me understand what is in your control that you intend to do well*

***Illogical* thinking**	If this happens, then that will surely follow. If I make a mistake, they will hold it against me for year	*Stop for a minute; and let's be logical here. What's your evidence they'll hold this against you for a year?*
***Blaming* thinking**	It's his fault. It's her fault. It's everyone's fault. It's not my fault!	*How possible could it be that actually it's nobody's fault? What's a more useful way to think about all this?*

We can see that by listening well to our own and others' language; looking out for any possible examples of unhelpful generalisations, deletions and distortions and, where appropriate, asking quality questions, we can seek to help ourselves and others to get a more balanced view of what's actually going on.

The power that our words have over us can be even greater than this, however. Have you ever found yourself in the company of someone and asked yourself questions such as: *What planet are they on?* or *I simply don't understand where you're coming from*. Sometimes, we need to listen so well to other people that we almost need to tune into their wavelength, and this is where we're going next.

Using language to tune into people

Up to about the 1970s, we used to have to tune in a radio to get on the right wavelength, so that we got the best signal. We can tune into people in a similar way.

In the 1980s, some ground breaking research by a Canadian psychologist called Shelle Rose Charvet revealed that there are some clear patterns in the way we all think and the language we use, which if we notice and tune into, can help enormously in increasing understanding and empathy between people.

As humans, we respond immediately when someone *speaks our language* and when we succeed in tuning into them. When people are tuned into each other and on the same wavelength, good things usually happen.

The kind of language that people use gives us clues about how they think; what motivates them and how they make decisions. If we can spot the patterns in the kind of language people use, we have a better chance of tuning into them, getting on their wavelength and thus having better quality conversations.

For example, have you noticed that some people tend to use language that is rather abstract and conceptual, while others tend to use language which is very specific, practical and grounded?

Likewise, some people focus more on, and talk more about, goals to be achieved. They may seem keen to manage priorities and are excited and energized by goals. In contrast, other people focus more on and talk about what should be avoided and got rid of and problems to be solved. Threats and deadlines energize them (they may even call targets *deadlines*).

Another pattern of thinking (and therefore language used) is where some people seem to like to make decisions based very much on their *internal* standards and values. They may take orders as information, and don't need praise or feedback. They provide their own motivation and judge the quality of their own work for themselves. They can become demotivated when they don't get to decide anything.

On the other hand, some people seem to prefer to pay more attention to what other people think and will use language that tells you they are doing this. These people are more likely to interpret information as orders and are motivated when someone else decides. They need outside feedback or results because they gather standards from the outside. In fact, they become demotivated and unsure of themselves in the absence of feedback. When they receive criticism or negative feedback, they question themselves.

Of course, as we engage with people and speak with and listen to them, it can at first be a challenge to begin to spot these patterns on what other people are focussing on and therefore speaking about, but the more we can spot these patterns the greater chance we have to tune into them and get on their wavelength.

A summary of some of the thinking patterns researched by Shelle Rose Charvet is below:

Thinking pattern	How to tune into people using this thinking pattern, and get onto their wavelength
The *Specific* thinking pattern People who prefer the *Specific* thinking pattern make up approx. 15% of the population. They need small pieces of sequential information. They may need to start over if the sequence is interrupted. They use lots of modifiers, adverbs and adjectives and speak in sequences step-by-step. They get frustrated with summaries and may have difficulty prioritizing.	To tune into people with this preference, seek to talk specifics with them, and listen to and appreciate the way they tend to like to tell a detailed story, rather than vague bigger picture concepts
The *Big Picture* thinking pattern	To tune into people with this preference, seek to talk to them about bigger picture

People who prefer the *Big Picture* thinking pattern make up approx 60% of the population. They prefer overviews and summaries, concepts and abstracts, and may present things in random order. They tend to use simple sentences with few modifiers or details, speaking in vague terms. Sometimes they don't specify the link between items and ideas, which can be confusing. They can get bored or feel overwhelmed with lots of detail. This pattern is useful when deciding on financial strategies, dealing with people and project management.	concepts, and listen to and enjoy their own explorations of open-ended possibilities and theories
The *Towards* thinking pattern People who prefer this thinking pattern make up approx 40% of the population. They consider goals to be achieved. They are good at managing priorities, and excited and energized by goals.	To tune into people with this preference, seek to talk to them about future aspirations they may have, their goals, and progress towards these. And listen to and enjoy their

They can have trouble considering potential obstacles.	own responses towards progress and future ambitions
The *Away From* thinking pattern People who prefer this thinking pattern make up approx 40% of the population. They consider what should be avoided; got rid of; and problems to be solved. Threats and deadlines energize them (they may call targets "deadlines"). They can be easily distracted, compelled to respond to negative situations, and can sometimes forget priorities and focus on the crisis	To tune into people with this preference, seek to talk to them about risks, problems, obstacles. And listen to and enjoy their own descriptions of deadlines met, and challenges, risks and obstacles met
The *Internal* thinking pattern People who prefer this pattern make up approx. 40% of the population. They gather information from the outside and decide based on internal standards. They take orders as information, and don't need praise or feedback. They provide	To tune into people with this preference, seek to talk about what's important to them as human beings, their values, their gut reaction to events and other people. And

their own motivation and judge the quality of their own work for themselves.	listen to and appreciate it when they speak more from the heart, possibly than the head.
The *External* thinking pattern	
People who prefer this thinking pattern make up approx 40% of the population. They are likely to interpret information as orders and are motivated when someone else decides. They need outside feedback or results because they gather standards from the outside. In fact, they become demotivated and unsure of themselves in the absence of feedback. When they receive criticism or negative feedback, they question themselves. (There's a group of about 20% of the population who seem comfortable using both of these thinking patterns equally)	To tune into people with this preference, seek to talk about the importance of seeking and acting on external feedback and external quality standards and kitemarks. And listen to and appreciate it when they talk about similar things
The *Options* thinking pattern	To tune into people with this preference,

People who prefer this thinking pattern make up approx. 40% of the population. They look for opportunities and possibilities. They create procedures and systems but don't follow them. They like breaking or bending the rules. They like starting things, development and setup. They don't like reducing their options.

When we ask: *Why did you choose?* they give a list of criteria. They are good at developing and testing safety procedures and process engineering. They are good at training design but not delivery. Unlimited choice motivates them.

The *Procedures* thinking pattern

People who prefer this thinking pattern make up approx 40% of the population. People who prefer this thinking pattern tend to believe there is a *right* way to do things. They are interested in seek to talk about new ideas and new ways of doing things, using creativity and starting new ideas running. And listen and appreciate it when they come up with new ideas of their own

To tune into people with this preference, seek to talk about the need for things to be done properly, in accordance with agreed procedures and

how to do things. They like to finish what they start. When you ask: *Why did you do it that way?* they give you a story or series of sequenced events, possibly referring to external rules or conventions. Anything to do with safety and security needs a person with this preference for this thinking pattern	commonly understood ways. Appreciate their views about things needing to be done properly

The next time you find yourself in a situation when the self-talk in your head says: *Why doesn't anyone listen to what I say or why can't they understand my point of view?* it may be that they use language differently from you. Pause, reflect and think what sort of language they're using and how you might be able to adapt your language to match theirs.

If you're interested in finding out more, there's a lot more information on this at:

https://www.labprofileonline.com/

Non-verbal communication

There's another form of communication that doesn't involve the spoken word: non-verbal communication. We all communicate constantly with our gestures, facial expressions and body language.

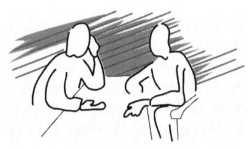

Public Domain Pictures[vii]

Research has shown that more than seventy percent of communication is non-verbal; and that we pick up subtle nuances of position, gesture and expression in our interactions with others. Furthermore, when we speak, others are as aware of rhythm, tone and inflection as they are of the words said. Even silence can sometimes speak volumes.

The initial research on this topic was conducted by Albert Mehrabian in the 1960s, who concluded that the following three elements account for communication:

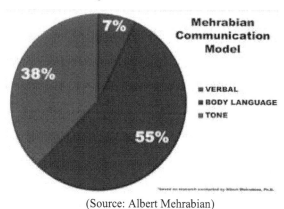

(Source: Albert Mehrabian)

There's a very amusing YouTube clip, called *Talking Eyebrows* which beautifully illustrates the power of non-verbal communication. Search YouTube on *Talking Eyebrows* and you can find out what we mean.

In this chapter, we've covered a lot of ground, including verbal and non-verbal communication; and how even silence can be used to communicate something. It's not surprising, therefore, is it, that we human beings often find ourselves misunderstood, or misunderstanding others – sometimes resulting in unfortunate (or worse) consequences in the world.

As Peter Drucker once said:

The most important thing about communication is noticing what's not being expressed
(https://succeedfeed.com)

And so, once again, as in chapter two, we realise the key importance of awareness; this time of our self-talk, the language we use with others, of the language others use with us and the subtle mix of non-verbal expression we and others use. Language is what we use when we're thinking so that is where we're going next. How useful would it be if we could understand more about the way we and others think? And so we progress onto the sixth Tool in our Happiness Toolkit: *Patterns of Thinking.*

Chapter nine: Patterns of thinking

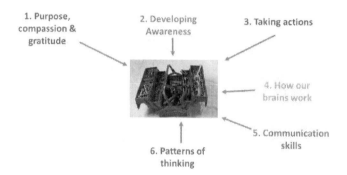

1. Purpose, compassion & gratitude
2. Developing Awareness
3. Taking actions
4. How our brains work
5. Communication skills
6. Patterns of thinking

We all think differently. We're all familiar with the idea that some people perceive situations with a *glass half full mindset* i.e. with optimism, and yet the same situation can be viewed with pessimism by a person using a *glass half empty mindset*. But it's probably true to say that the fact that we all think differently isn't as well understood as it might be, and over the history of mankind this fact possibly explains why there has been such unhappiness, warfare and human misery amongst our species.

That's why in this chapter, we're devoting our attention to various aspects of thinking differently, expanding the ways we each think and appreciating and valuing different thinking styles from our own which support our understanding of ourselves and others.

Have a look at the picture below. What do you notice most?

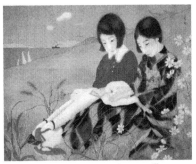

Public Domain Pictures[viii]

We've asked this question dozens of times in workshops, and we invariably find that about half of the group say something such as *a Japanese picnic on the beach*; and the other half typically say something such as *two ladies reading a book*; *four lovely open toe sandals*; and *boats out at sea*. Typically, then, some people start questioning each other – with a degree of confusion and surprise – to seek to understand how other people noticed what they noticed, quickly followed by some laughter and a series of *ahaa* moments!

What does this show? It's an example of how some people think in a way which focusses on the "big picture" – the overall impression. Whereas, if our minds are directed towards looking at the detail, this style of thinking can result in us noticing entirely different things.

There are two important points which help to enhance the quality of our lives. Firstly, understanding, appreciating and valuing different thinking styles in both ourselves and others and secondly, being able to flex our own thinking styles and adopt new ones. That's the main theme of the rest of this chapter.

It can help when we understand our own preferred thinking style.

Thinking Styles

Much of our thinking comes from habits, or patterns we've used possibly for years: some of them might even have been shaped by our parents or other close relatives. Here's a short questionnaire based on the work of Ed Diener (2008), which gives us a flavour of some habitual patterns of thinking we may currently have. Being aware of what we currently do, can give us a platform to celebrate any patterns of thinking that serve us well, or to consider if there's anything we might want to change. This questionnaire may give you an insight into your own thinking style.

Thinking Styles Questionnaire

For each item, simply assign a "1" if you think it is broadly true for you.

Thinking Pattern A

Most people will take advantage of you if you give them the slightest chance	
When something bad happens, I tend to dwell on it for a long time	
When I think of the past, for some reason, bad things usually stand out	
I often regret many things from my past	
I think frequently about opportunities I have missed	
I frequently compare myself to others	
When I see others prosper, it can make me feel bad about myself	
When good things happen, I often wonder if they might have been even better	
When good things happen, I often wonder if they will soon turn sour	
When somebody does something for me, I often wonder if they have an ulterior motive	
When I think of myself, I usually think of my many shortcomings	
I see my community as a place full of problems	

I quickly notice the mistakes others make	
I often see the faults in others	
TOTAL:	

Thinking Pattern B

I think it's good to be generous in expressing my appreciation to others for what they do	
I am usually optimistic about the positive difference I can make the world	
I usually see many opportunities in the world	
I know the world has its problems, but it seems like a wonderful place overall	
I usually notice the little good things others do	
When I see others prosper, even strangers, I am usually happy for them	
I often savour memories of pleasant past times	
When I think of the past, the happy times usually come to my mind most	
I sometimes think how fortunate I have been in my life	
When something bad happens, I often see a "silver lining"	

I usually see myself as a person with many strengths	
I believe in the good qualities of other people	
I usually see the good in most people	
I usually see much beauty around me	
TOTAL:	

There are 2 thinking styles here. Thinking Pattern A tends towards seeing the glass half empty, whereas Thinking Patten B tends towards seeing the glass half full. (But it's the same glass of course). Each of these thinking styles has its use, its pros and cons. You might want to reflect on which thinking style is your preference and how well is serves you, and in what contexts. It can also be instructive and fun to compare your scores with others.

In chapter seven, we quoted Prof Sir Robin Murray, who once said:

The brain is the most complex thing in the universe

Each of us probably only uses a tiny fraction of this fantastic organ in our heads. How wonderful it would be if we could all say that we use our brains to make us brilliant thinkers and use those grey cells to their full potential. That's where we're going next. We're going to explore the best things that brilliant thinkers do and see how we can do more of this ourselves.

How to Think Brilliantly

On her website, Susan Singam tells the famous story of the corpse that bleeds:

A psychiatrist was treating a man who believed he was a corpse. Despite all the psychiatrist's logical arguments, the man persisted in his belief. In a flash of inspiration, the psychiatrist asked the man. "Do corpses bleed?" The patient replied: "That's ridiculous. Of course corpses don't bleed." After first asking for permission, the psychiatrist pricked the man's finger and produced a drop of bright red blood. The patient looked at his bleeding finger with astonishment and exclaimed: "I'll be damned, corpses do bleed!"

http://human-equation.com/do-corpses-bleed/)

We can see how important it is to be aware of how we think and of how our thoughts create our own personal version of reality. Brilliant thinkers recognise there are many different views of the world – and that each one is incomplete. Einstein once said: *Imagination is more important than knowledge.* What he meant was that it's important to be able to flex our brains so that we can think in lots of different ways, i.e. to think brilliantly.

Brilliant thinkers do a number of things well, including:

- knowing their preferred thinking styles, others' thinking styles, and appreciate and value them all
- challenging assumptions
- incubating ideas and possibilities
- being resilient in overcoming obstacles and bouncing back from adversity

Let's take each of these in turn.

Knowing our preferred thinking styles, others' thinking styles, and appreciating and valuing them all

Our brain is divided into two halves, or hemispheres, that are connected to each other by the corpus callosum. These two hemispheres control the motion in and receive sensory inputs from the opposite side of our body. In other words, the left hemisphere controls the right side of our body and receives sensory inputs from the right side of our body.

The left hemisphere of our brain handles tasks such as reading, writing, speaking, arithmetic reasoning and understanding. Studies shows that when we speak or do arithmetic calculations, activity increases in our left hemisphere. Another characteristic of our left hemisphere is that it tends to process information sequentially, one at a time.

The right hemisphere of our brain excels in visual perception, understanding spatial relationships, recognizing patterns, music, emotional expressions, etc. It's also good at making inferences. For example, when primed with words such as *foot, cry* and *glass* our right hemisphere will relate these words to *cut*.

Our left hemisphere knows all these words individually but is unable to quickly make inferences from them. Our right hemisphere also lets us perceive the sense of self. People with lesions in the right brain sometimes have difficulty recognizing themselves in the mirror. Unlike the left hemisphere, our right hemisphere tends to process information as a whole.

In the same sense that most of us have a preferred hand to write with, most of us have a preference for whether, and to what extent, we think using the left or the right-hand side of the brain.

In the 1990s, Dr Geil Browning and Wendell Williams dedicated themselves to researching and creating a psychometric tool with strict database management that adults could use which valued the diversity of how we all think and behave. They committed to preserve the statistical validity of their model and keep it current with human brain research. They discovered there are four different Thinking Styles that we all have access to, and they called their model of thinking and behaving *Emergenetics*.

The 4 Emergenetics Thinking Styles are:

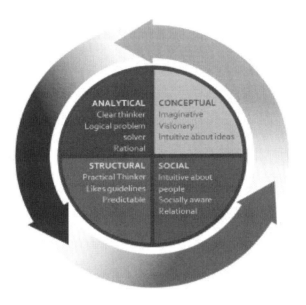

Geil Browning's research shows that there a few people in the world who prefer pretty much to use all four Thinking Styles equally; but for most of us, we prefer to think with one or more of the Thinking Styles.

On many occasions, we will be in the company of people who think differently. Those who think in a similar way are often people we get on well with, and those who think differently are, conversely, people we may find more of a challenge. More details of each of the four Thinking Styles that emerged from Geil Browning's research are described below:

Patterns of thinking

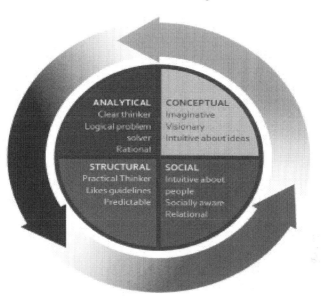

Analytical Thinkers ask questions such as:	Conceptual Thinkers ask questions such as:
<ul><li>Why?</li><li>How do you know that? What are the facts?</li><li>Where is the logic here?</li></ul>	<ul><li>What if?</li><li>Can I try this new idea on you?</li><li>How could this be different in the future?</li></ul>
Structural Thinkers ask questions such as:	**Social Thinkers ask questions such as:**
<ul><li>What are the practical applications?</li></ul>	<ul><li>Who's involved in this?</li></ul>

• What are the next steps? • What's the plan? • What are the risks and how can we manage them?	• What do others think? • How can we involve others in this?

Understanding our own thinking preferences and others' preferences is important in order to get the best out of each other.

Here's a short quiz to help you get a handle on each Thinking Style (the answers are in the Appendix at the back of the book).

	Statement	Which Thinking Style is this?
1	What are the facts here?	
2	How do other people feel about this?	
3	What are the next steps?	
4	Imagine how this could change the future	
5	I need to ask how this fits with our values	
6	How practical is all this?	
7	I wonder what new opportunities this creates for us?	

8	Logically, this makes no sense	
9	What's the missing information here?	
10	What's the correct procedure for this?	
11	What would others expect from us?	
12	Just imagine the new options this opens up	

The Emergenetics model is the result of rigorous and extensive research into people's preferences of thinking and behaving; is soundly based in neuroscience and is a powerful way to enhance our flexibility in how we think and behave. Emergenetics is used extensively by coaches and in organisations to unleash the full potential of individuals, teams and organisations, by making people more aware of their natural preferences and by giving them more choices in thinking and behaving. If you're interested in getting a full personal profile and personal feedback, you can take the full Emergenetics questionnaire by contacting:

https://www.emergenetics.com/uk/take_a_profile/

Understanding our own and others' thinking preferences is so important, especially when we as individuals or as a society need to go back to the fundamentals of how we want or need to live our lives. As we all know, the Covid-19 experience has made us all question whether and to what extent we can or should return to the *old normal*; or whether we now have an opportunity to construct *a new and better normal*. In other words, as we stand at this crossroads, we need more than ever to think creatively about what we want from and with life, and to do this, we need to draw on as much quality thinking as possible. A curious aspect of humanity is that we tend to prefer to surround ourselves with people who think like us – this makes us more comfortable somehow. But the downside of this is that we can get groupthink and miss opportunities. Use of the Emergenetics Thinking Styles is an excellent way to make sure we tick all the boxes and get as much rich thinking as possible.

Challenging assumptions

Another key to brilliant thinking is the ability to ask great questions; and in so doing, to challenge assumptions. By using all of the four Thinking Styles described above, we can significantly increase the range of good quality questions we ask, and brilliant thinking happens when we use these great questions to challenge commonly held assumptions. Edward de Bono (1985) describes this skill as "lateral thinking", and for him, this is largely about asking great questions to challenge what he calls "dominant ideas", i.e. commonly held beliefs about how the world works and how things should be done. There are dominant ideas in every walk of life. They are the assumptions, rules and conventions that underpin people's and society's thinking and attitudes. For hundreds of years, mankind thought the earth was flat and that the Earth was the centre of the universe.

One of the best quality questions to ask which can challenge dominant ideas is *What if...?* But to make this question work well, we also need to make sure that it's asked at the right time, and in the right context – not when everyone is late for lunch and stressed out!

Another useful tool to help challenge dominant ideas is the use of humour (again at the right time and in the right context). Humour is helpful in seeing things in new ways. It also releases endorphins which can relieve tension and make people feel better.

Finally, another important aspect of challenging assumptions is to build quiet reflection into our daily/weekly routine (ideally regularly, so that the brain gets used to it). The following four reflection questions, used regularly, are very helpful:

1	*What happened and why did it happen in this way?*
2	*How did I think and feel about what happened?*
3	*What did I learn from this experience?*
4	*What will I change (behaviours, attitudes, thoughts and feelings) as a result of this learning?*

A regular habit of quality reflection leads into the next key part of brilliant thinking, incubation and the use of sleep.

<u>Incubating ideas and possibilities</u>

Creativity is one of the most important assets we have to navigate through the fast changing world of the 21st century. Often, creative discoveries result from a process whereby initial *conscious thought* is followed by a period of quiet, *unconscious mulling*. Almost as if the person concerned delegates the issue to the unconscious mind. They might say something like: *I'm not sure – let me sleep on it.* And then, one finds the solution or a new angle on the issue suddenly popping into consciousness while taking a shower.

In addition, it's important to value the role that sleep plays in creative thinking. For example, Paul McCartney announced in the 1960s that he came up with the melody for *Yesterday* in a dream and the Nobel Prize winner Loewi woke up with the idea for how to prove his theory of chemical neurotransmission.

The explanation here is that the brain has specific brain wave patterns, each of which is associated with specific mental functions:

In chapter seven, we covered some of the main changes that happen in our brains when we go to sleep. Here's a reminder of the different brain wave patterns associated with sleep:

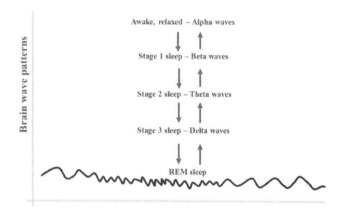

A typical good night's sleep consists of a number of repeated cycles each lasting about ninety minutes, when the brain waves shift from the Alpha wave pattern, through the Theta wave pattern, down through the Delta wave pattern, into the Rapid Eyeball Movement (REM) phase, and then back up to the Alpha wave pattern again.

People who think brilliantly understand that the brain needs to do this, and that overnight, they can get major new hunches and ideas which they might well have *scratched their head about* the previous day, using their conscious mind. They also understand the brain's need to do this well; first of which is to keep regular sleeping hours. This programmes the brain and internal body clock to get used to a set routine.

We also know from chapter seven that good quality sleep improves our immune system, thus making us more resilient to help us bounce back from adversity.

Being resilient in overcoming obstacles and bouncing back from adversity

Someone once said: *You don't drown by falling in the water. You drown by staying there.* Brilliant thinkers have the mental agility and skill to find their way out of the water, once they have fallen into it. In other words, to bounce back from adversity well. So, what thinking tools and techniques do brilliant thinkers use to achieve this?

Also in chapter seven, we refer to the key importance of listening to our self-talk (that loop of constant chatter in our head – much of which can be unhelpful). The tone of our self-talk, repeated frequently in our heads, shapes our attitudes to life – our mindset, if you like. A non-resilient mindset may contain some or all of the following elements:

Non Resilient Mindset

"Oh no, I've just made another mistake..."

• This ruins everything..	PERVASIVE
• I'll never get anywhere now..	PERMANENT
• Just shows how useless I am..	PERSONAL

On the other hand, the kinds of things a brilliant thinker (and resilient person) will say to themselves are:

Resilient Mindset

"Oh no, I've just made another mistake…"

• What must I do differently..	**LEARNING**
• I need to get more feedback..	**ACTION**
• It's down to me to do better..	**ACCOUNTABLE**

In other words, a brilliant thinker and resilient person will have a different internal mental landscape, based on learning, action and personal accountability. Another way of understanding resilience is to see the links with emotional intelligence. We deal more with this topic in chapter ten, where we refer to the research work of Jo Maddocks and Dan Hughes (2019). Their research shows a clear link between these five factors and the ability to bounce back from adversity:

- having a strong sense of inner confidence
- adopting an optimistic but realistic perspective
- having a clear sense of purpose
- regulating emotions and not over-reacting
- taking personal responsibility for what happens to oneself

Finally, in his *Seven Habits* book, Steven Covey has a useful model called *Circles of Concern* which contributes enormously to resilience and good quality thinking:

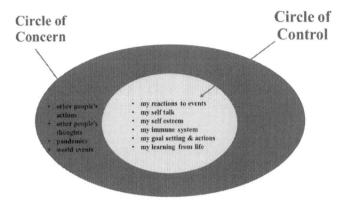

The key here of course, is to focus our mind on the things that are in our own control (or influence); and not to waste energy, thoughts and precious time on things that are outside our control (or influence). There is one more important part of resilience. This concerns how strong we are internally to resist and deal with unwanted infections: the strength of our personal immune system.

Our immune systems

If we pause for a moment and think about the words or phrases we've most often heard from experts or politicians about the Covid-19 initial lockdown period (or subsequently), what comes to mind most readily? Maybe you might think of words such as:

- furlough
- protect the NHS
- PPE
- two metres social distancing

- social isolation
- following the science
- underlying health conditions
- stay alert

One term we cannot recall hearing being used on the media is our *immune system*, and we find this surprising, since, surely this, a key part of our personal resilience, is one aspect of our health and well-being that for most of us at least, is in our control. If we choose a lifestyle which doesn't allow our personal immune system to flourish, how likely is it that we can be fully happy and fulfilled – since we won't be at our best, and possibly prone to lots of illnesses.

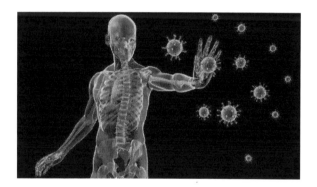

Humans have a multi-layered defence thanks to a network formed by the lymphatic system, specifically designed organs (e.g. spleen and thymus gland) and circulating cells and proteins. There are other defence mechanisms:

- skin: our skin provides a great barrier (unless you have cuts or abrasions)

- bugs: bugs that enter the nose trigger cells to make more protective mucus
- sneezing: sneezes and coughs force invading microbes out
- stomach acid: acid in our stomach destroys pathogens that you swallow
- gut lining: our gut has a whole mucosal defence team onboard
- tiny hairs: small hairs in the airways known as cilia keep mucus moving to remove infections

But probably the greatest defence available to us is our personal immune system. The US National Institute of Health defines this system as *a network of cells, tissues, and organs that work together to defend the body against attacks by external invaders. These are primarily microbes (germs)— tiny, infection-causing organisms such as bacteria, viruses, parasites, and fungi.* Because the human body provides an ideal environment for many microbes, they try to break in. It's the immune system's job to keep them out or, failing that, to seek out and destroy them.

During the Covid-19 pandemic, yet another phrase we have often heard, quite rightly, is *unsung heroes*; and our personal immune system is probably the greatest unsung hero of all. When it's working well, of course, most of us take it for granted, but when it struggles to cope with a new disease, we quite understandably go into crisis mode. How many times have we heard ourselves or others say something like: *I'm feeling a bit run down,* which means that our bodies are telling us we need to rest a bit more, and get our immune system stronger. We all know what can happen when we're feeling run down: it leaves us vulnerable to colds, coughs, flu, and perhaps from now on, to Covid-19 or other coronaviruses. Our personal immune system is a bit like our own personal knight in shining white armour. The horse, the armour, the shield are all important for our survival, but they are no use at all if we don't have the inner physical, biological and mental resilience to ride the horse, to wear the armour and to wield the sword.

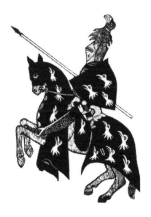

Good Free Photos[ix]

Maybe one of the aspects of the new normal, as we learn to live with the new reality, is that we will all need to pay more attention to developing our personal immune system more. We've already seen in chapter seven how good sleep habits are important to help our immune systems repair and strengthen themselves, and this takes us to the wider issue of our lifestyles. Scientists still do not have a perfect understanding of exactly how our immune systems work, but common sense alone, plus the concept of showing compassion to ourselves others and the world points to the need for us all, in addition to getting enough quality sleep, to:

- avoid smoking
- eat a diet high in fruits and vegetables
- exercise regularly
- maintain a healthy weight
- drink in moderation
- balance stress well with adequate recovery

There are lots of sources of scientific research on the immune system, and one of the most useful is Harvard Health at:

https://www.health.harvard.edu/staying-healthy/how-to-boost-your-immune-system

In addition to the things we can do ourselves to strengthen our personal immune system, it's becoming increasingly clear that the quality of the environment we live in has a big impact on the quality of our immune system. No doubt, the Covid-19 pandemic will be the subject of scientific research for years to come, but there are already some interesting findings. For example, the pandemic has shown that pollution lowers our resistance to disease. More exposure to traffic fumes means weaker lungs and greater risk of dying from Covid-19, according to scientists at Harvard University. In other words, could it be that our current lifestyles and their associated pollution levels have made us more vulnerable to Covid-19, or even created the conditions for the virus to spread to humans in the first place? If so, perhaps we should be exploring what social and economic conditions need to be in place to prevent the virus spread, rather than simply locking down, and expecting to return to normal as it used to be?

Even so, there are probably few people in the Western world who could hand on heart say that their lifestyle is one hundred percent conducive to a strong immune system, and it could be worthwhile considering this question:

> *What's the smallest and most significant change I could make to my lifestyle, which I could make a personal habit and which would help boost my immune system, thus making me more resilient?*

In our lives, we seem to need strength to overcome so many kinds of obstacles. Another common obstacle which we all face from time to time, and for which we need resilience to bounce back from are the times when we ourselves, or other people whose company we share, have a bad mood, feel stressed or irritable. This takes us nicely into the next section which adds a little more brain science to the topic.

Mood contagion

Have you ever noticed how if a group of people are in the same room, and a new person enters the room happens to have a different mood (happier or gloomier) from everyone else in the room, that it's almost as if the overall mood of the room changes to become more like the mood of the new person?

Well, there is now some research which explains how this (mood contagion) happens.

In the last thirty years or so, researchers have made a fascinating discovery about the brain. A set of neurons in the brain exist, known as *mirror neurons*. A mirror neuron is a brain cell that fires both when an animal does something and when the animal observes the same action performed by another.

These neurons are theorized to be partly responsible for explaining how humans and monkeys can imitate behaviour. The discovery of mirror neurons occurred in an Italian laboratory where the brains of rhesus monkeys were linked up to electrodes, and their brains' neuronal activity was monitored. One of the scientists noticed that some regions of the brain became active in the monkeys who were watching him. Further investigation showed that these same regions lit up in the monkeys when they were eating or watching somebody else eat and that they correlated both with the motion of holding food as well as the feeling of being hungry.

Thus, *mirror neurons* in the brains of primates and humans were discovered.

Elaine Hatfield, a co-author of a pioneering academic book *Emotional Contagion* and a professor of psychology at the University of Hawaii, defines *primitive* emotional contagion as the *tendency to automatically mimic and synchronize facial expressions, vocalizations, postures, and movements with those of another person and, consequently, to converge emotionally.* Primitive emotional contagion is a basic building block of human interaction. It helps us coordinate and synchronize with others, empathize with them, and read their minds—all critical survival skills. Her research shows that intense negative emotions that are expressed more emphatically are more contagious.

Positive, emotional contagion can be a wonderful thing. But at times such as those associated with Covid-19, it's possible to become infected by the negative emotions of those in our circle of friends, our family at home, our colleagues, the people we follow on social media or the news. What's been happening recently is that some of us have been catching the anxiety around us and transferring it to others, who have been relaying it back to us, in an almost perpetual cycle of negative emotion. Our isolation can also be dispiriting, and lead to social loneliness, which can have a debilitating effect on our mood and happiness, and which in turn makes us even more susceptible to negative emotional contagion. And although emotions are more contagious in person, they can still be transmitted and caught online – by phone, email, or any other remote interaction with other people. This is why it's so important for us to be aware of how we're responding to our surroundings and our situations at the moment, and how we're reacting to emotional contagion, even while we're at home.

This comes down to awareness. Understanding how emotional contagion works increases our awareness of the negative version of it, and this can prevent the spread of anxiety and worry that we're seeing. It's reasonable to feel some fear and worry, but understanding how negative emotional contagion works can help us navigate through this period.

How can we manage negative emotions at the moment? We can stay away from places or people that exacerbate our feelings of worry and panic. Maybe limit our social media time, or the amount of time we're watching the news. And if we're watching the news, or reading from news sources, make sure we're getting information from legitimate sources and experts. Find ways to share with others, show kindness, volunteer if you can, exercise regularly, and engage in high quality connections with others – even if this is online. All of these things will enhance positive feelings and increase your mood. Feelings of hope have been shown to be more important than feelings of fear when it comes to being resilient against poor outcomes, and purposefully expressing optimism and gratitude are important triggers for long-term well-being. We need this positivity to counterbalance the swirling negative emotions resulting from the Covid -19 pandemic. In other words, we each have a responsibility each day to take at least one simple action to be happier, and help others to be happier, even if it's just a smile or a random act of kindness.

We've covered a lot of territory in this chapter about patterns of thinking: but then again, that's understandable since there's so much there. Without doubt, the more we can begin to understand the key aspects of that miraculous muscle between our ears, the more success we'll have in our lives and the happier we'll be. Now, armed with this knowledge of patterns of thinking, we're going onto the seventh Tool in our Happiness Toolkit, which is about understanding more about personality and relationships.

Chapter ten: Understanding personality and relationships

And now, we move onto one of the most important ways to understand ourselves and others – the seventh Tool in our Happiness toolkit: *understanding personality and relationships*:

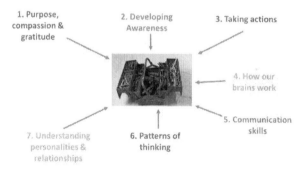

1. Purpose, compassion & gratitude

2. Developing Awareness

3. Taking actions

4. How our brains work

5. Communication skills

6. Patterns of thinking

7. Understanding personalities & relationships

At least since the time of Ancient Greece, people have been intrigued by the concept of personality. In 370 BC, Hippocrates proposed a model of *temperaments* according to which some people's personalities were linked to specific temperaments. Plato suggested that people's personalities were a mixture of four factors (artistic, intuitive, sensible and reasoning).

Today, we often describe and assess the personalities of the people around us. *She has such a great personality,* you might say about a friend. *He gets his personality from his dad* you might say about your son. Since the concept of personality is so commonplace, let's now seek to understand it a bit more.

Research on personality is well established and has led to the development of a number of theories and models that help explain how and why certain personality traits develop. There are various models of personality to choose from, including FIRO B, Insights, DISC, the Enneagram and Thomas International to name a few. Any internet search will reveal a host more. One of the most respected is called the Myers Briggs Type Indicator and it's this that we want to explore now.

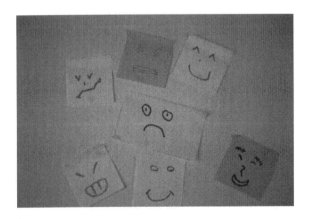

The Myers Briggs Type Indicator (MBTI)

In the 1930s - 1940s, an American mother and daughter, Katharine Cook Briggs and Isabel Briggs Myers researched extensively the recurring patterns they noticed in human behaviours, resulting in the development of the Myers-Briggs Type Indicator (MBTI). The research resulted in 1980 in the publication of *Gifts Differing.* It's probably the most enduring and most widely used ever of all the models of personality. It's underpinned by the theories of Carl Jung, the Swiss psychologist. The MBTI is frequently used in the areas of teaching and academia, group dynamics, employee training, leadership training, marriage counselling, and personal development.

The more insight we have about our personality and that of others, the more chance we have to flex our thinking, emotions and actions to get the best of ourselves and of our relationships. In that sense, the Myers-Briggs Type Indicator (MBTI) can yield much personal change and growth.

Although you can find out more from various websites, we've included here for you a brief overview:

Some people seem to prefer talking a lot; but others seem to prefer to listen

Extraversion–Introversion (E–I)

The Extraversion – Introversion (E – I) scale is designed to reflect whether a person is an extravert or an introvert in the manner described by Jung. He regarded extraversion and introversion as *mutually complementary* attitudes whose differences *generate the tension that both the individual and society need for the maintenance of life.* Extraverts are oriented primarily toward the outer world, thus they tend to focus their perception and judgment on people and objects. Introverts are oriented primarily toward their inner world.

> **Some people seem to prefer to focus more on the detail; but others seem to prefer to focus on the bigger picture**

Sensing–Intuition (S–N)

The Sensing – Intuition (S-N) scale is designed to reflect a person's preference between two opposite ways of perceiving. Some people rely primarily upon the process of sensing (S), which reports observable facts or happenings through one or more of the five senses (taste, sight, touch, smell and hearing.). Other people rely first and foremost on the process of intuition (N), which is all about the bigger picture, meanings, relationships and/or possibilities that have been worked out beyond the reach of the conscious mind.

> **Some people seem to prefer to focus more on logic; but others seem to prefer to focus on how they and others feel**

Thinking–Feeling (T–F)

The Thinking – Feeling (T – F) scale is designed to reflect a person's preference between two contrasting ways of making decisions. Some people rely primarily on the use of objective logic to make decisions, through Thinking (T) to decide issues impersonally. Other people rely more on a more subjective way to make decisions, based on values, and feelings. This is a process known as Feeling (F).

Some people prefer structure in their lives: whereas other people prefer more spontaneity

Judging – Perceiving (J – P)

The Judging – Perceiving (J – P) scale is designed to describe the process used primarily in dealing with the outer world, that is, with the *extraverted* part of life. A person who prefers Judgment (J) has a preference for using a Judgment process (either Thinking or Feeling) for dealing with the outer world. A person who prefers Perception (P) has a preference for using a Perception process (either Sensing or Intuition) for dealing with the outer world.

Summary of the Types

Given the above, after someone has completed the MBTI questionnaire and had it fed back by a qualified practitioner, the person taking the questionnaire uses the results of the questionnaire and the feedback to review their preferences for each of the Types below:

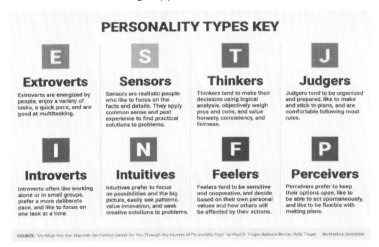

This produces a mixture of four types, such as someone who prefers for example:

- ESTJ (Extroversion, Sensing, Thinking, Judging), or
- INFP (Introversion, Intuition, Feeling, Perceiving)

Finally, a cautionary note about how the tool is sometimes used. The MBTI is all about how we *prefer* to behave. Just as most of are blessed with two hands and have a preference to use one of these to write with, we can, if we choose (and practice enough), use our other hand to write with. In the same way, it's important that we don't limit and stereotype ourselves by reference to our four MBTI letters. For example, a person who has a preference for Extraversion (E) also has available to them the gifts of Introversion, and ditto for the other three aspects of the model. In fact, one could say that the identification of the preferred types is just the starting point of personal development – as we embark on learning how to use the gifts and talents of the *opposite* four letters: a life long journey.

You may already know your MBTI type, or you may have a hunch how it would come out if you did the questionnaire. If you would like to do the questionnaire, you can do so using this link:

https://eu.themyersbriggs.com/en/tools/MBTI/MBTI-Step-I

The Emergenetics Profile

We mentioned in chapter nine, a well respected and well researched tool to give us insights into how we and others tend to think and behave, called *Emergenetics*. This tool is soundly based in neuroscience and is a powerful way to enhance our flexibility in how we think and behave. Emergenetics has been used extensively by coaches and in organisations. It comes with a very useful app, which means it's easy to remind ourselves of our own personal profile, and the profiles of others too, if they've given their agreement to share theirs with us.

The full Emergenetics profile provides much more than a description of our preferred Thinking Styles. It also provides a subtle description of some key behavioural preferences; and gives us a powerful picture of personality, and our potential to flex and develop that personality. The Emergenetics profiles also have the added bonus of comparing our personal results with the global population, so that we can see at a glance how similar or different we are to most other people. If you would like to take a full profile, you can do so by contacting its website:

https://www.emergenetics.com/uk/take_a_profile/

Archetypes: Discovering Unconscious Patterns

In chapter seven, we explored the role of the *unconscious mind* in driving our thoughts, emotions and actions, and this was one of the greatest insights that the Swiss psychologist, Carl Jung bequeathed us. Much of the delight and the frustration of being human is that there is always more to our inner world than we can ever imagine. Have you, for example, ever found yourself asking questions such as:

- *why did I do that….again!?*
- *why do I keep ending up in the same situation?*
- *who is the perfect life partner for me?*
- *what kind of job would I really like?*

At one time or another, most of us find ourselves ask ourselves questions like these. Such questions are usually easier than their answers. We don't always know why we do what we do: probably because so much of what we think, do and feel is driven by our unconscious mind.

Carl Jung observed a number of patterns which occur at an unconscious level: which he called *archetypes.* He proposed that people go through life drawing from a repertoire of instinctive roles: father, mother, child, lover, creator, warrior, caregiver, and an untold number of others. Jung claimed there are as many archetypes *as there are typical situations in life.* Each of us is capable of playing any one of these countless characters at any time in the stories of our lives. Yet, out of the countless archetypal roles available, each of us uses a select few more frequently than others. These are called our *dominant archetypes.* Often the characteristics of a dominant archetype fit a particular situation or challenge. But sometimes we're like the proverbial hammer that sees only nails, applying the same solution even when the situation demands a different approach. We can be blind to other options lurking outside our usual attention, often operating unconsciously. In extreme cases, the resulting self-deception or lack of self-knowledge may be harmful:

> **There is no lunacy people under**
> **the domination of an archetype**
> **will not fall prey to**
> (Jung, 1959)

Identifying which archetypes are influential in our lives can thus lead us to self-discovery, self-awareness, growth, and self-actualization. Consciously choosing the right archetype for each chapter in our life story can create a more fulfilling, successful life, where we use our archetypes instead of being controlled by them.

The Center for Applications of Psychological Type, Inc. (CAPT®) offers a scientifically validated assessment instrument, available online, that measures archetypes and brings their unconscious influence to our awareness.

The Pearson Marr Archetype Indicator (PMAI®) assessment, created by Carol Pearson and Hugh Marr, is designed for use by individuals. Personal reports show the relative influence of twelve archetypal patterns in our life.

Archetype	Description of the archetype's gifts
Innocent	Developing the trust, confidence & optimism to do the life journey
Orphan	Recognising that bad things happen, and developing realism and resilience
Warrior	Learning to compete, set goals and when necessary, defend oneself
Caregiver	Showing care, concern & compassion for others
Seeker	Being willing to be different, having the courage to try new things
Lover	Loving others, being romantic intimate & making commitments
Destroyer	Letting go & starting over, taking action to end bad situations
Creator	Demonstrating imagination, innovation & cleverness
Ruler	Taking charge, being responsible, living according to your values
Magician	Changing what happens by altering your own thoughts & behaviours
Sage	Thinking clearly, critically & formulating your own opinions

Jester	Enjoying your life and your work. Being here now

It's almost as if our unconscious mind has twelve characters or energies at its disposal, to be used throughout our lives. Each archetype brings with it certain characteristic energy and gifts, as can be seen in the above table. Carol Pearson has a website which provides lots more information and insights about her model and this can be found at:

www.storywell.com

Each stage of our life may justify or need more or less use of a particular archetype. For example, a young person about to leave school and enter the adult world will probably want more of the energy of the:

- Warrior
- Lover
- Seeker
- Creator

But this same young person may also need to be able to use the gifts of the Destroyer archetype, to be able to move away from home and family successfully. If we're trying to change from old patterns of behaviour to different ones, it may be that the Destroyer archetype is particularly important. As someone moves into late adulthood, possibly as a grandparent, they may want to bring other archetypes more into play such as the Sage, Magician and Jester.

The twelve archetypes naturally cluster into three groupings, as shown below, and it can be valuable to stop, pause and reflect in life and review which archetypes are most and least prevalent in one's life; and if the balance needs to change in any way.

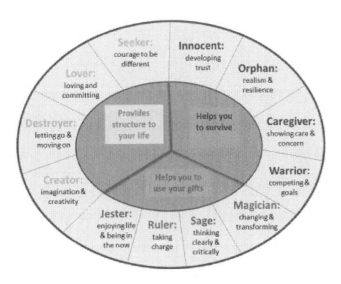

CAPT's archetype assessment instrument, the Pearson Marr Archetype Indicator (PMAI®) costs about £15 to take on line, recognizes the importance of archetypes and provides an easy to read and understanding of which archetypes might be most and least active in one's life.

https://www.capt.org/catalog/Archetype-Assessment-Personal.htm

Archetypes link to our unconscious. Assessing archetypal influence, therefore, can provide an avenue to a deeper level of self-awareness and understanding of others. Awareness allows us to intentionally write our life story to be the best it can be. The accompanying online workbook provides guidance in consciously deciding which archetypes to use, when to use them, and which to develop.

Finally, the guidance about the PMAI instrument also alerts us to the potential consequences of over-using certain archetypes, or using them with ill intent or with low skills: as can be seen below:

Archetype	Description of the archetype's potential downsides
Innocent	Naivety, childish dependence
Orphan	Cynicism, tendency to be victim
Warrior	Arrogance, ruthlessness
Caregiver	Martyrdom, co-dependence
Seeker	Inability to commit, alienation
Lover	Objectifying others, using people as things
Destroyer	Doing harm to self or others
Creator	Self indulgence, creating messes, prima donna
Ruler	Rigidity, controlling behaviours
Magician	Manipulation of others
Sage	Being overly critical, pomposity, know it all
Jester	Cruelty, debauchery, con artistry

There are times in life, when we sometimes face stiff challenges, such as having to summon up courage to deal with a difficult relationship, to stand our ground against a bully, or to show care to someone in distress. In such circumstances, knowing about the Pearson Marr Archetypes Indicator (PMAI) can help us to draw on the internal resources we need to deal with the situation, and overcome the obstacles we face.

And, as we say above, there's always more to understand about our inner worlds. In this spirit, we now move onto the inspirational work of a Canadian psychiatrist, Eric Berne, who in the 1950s and 1960s, focussed more on understanding the interactions between people, and the recurring patterns that his research revealed. In the action planning that you'll have done as a result of the earlier chapters, you may have sometimes found that you encounter obstacles in the implementation of your plans and involves your relationship with one or more people. Often, there can be underlying reasons why the obstacles occur and even recur. The work of Eric Berne can help us enormously to understand and remove the obstacles.

Relationships

Have you ever met anyone who is constantly critical, and often wanting to put you (and the rest of the world) right? Have you ever been with anyone who you think is patronising to you? Someone who treats you as if you were a child?

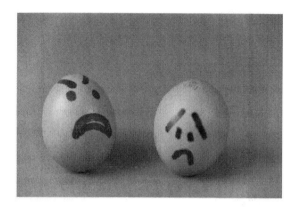

Well, here is yet another set of patterns in human behaviour which often get in the way of effective relationships, both in family and in work life. It's called Transactional Analysis and focuses on the interactions between people when they exhibit behaviours found when we're in the roles of parent, adult or child.

Transactional Analysis: Parent, Adult, Child

Based on his observations of people in his own clinical practice in the 1950s, the psychologist Eric Berne developed the idea in his ground breaking book *Games People Play* (1960) that people can switch between different states of mind—sometimes in the same conversation and certainly in different parts of their lives, for example at work and at home. He summarised these states of mind into three types of thinking which he called:

- Parent
- Adult
- Child

The **Child** state consists of parts of ourselves which hark back to our childhood. It is childlike but not childish. In this state *reside intuition, creative and spontaneous drive and enjoyment.* When we're in the Child state, we act like the child we once were. We aren't just putting on an act; we think, feel, see, hear and react as a three or five or eight-year-old child.

When the Child is hateful or loving, impulsive, spontaneous or playful it's called the *Natural Child.* When it's thoughtful, creative or imaginative it's called the *Little Professor.* When it's fearful, guilty or ashamed, it's called the *Adapted Child.* The Child has all the feelings; fear, love, anger, joy, sadness, shame and so on. The Child is often blamed for being the source of people's troubles because it's self-centred, emotional, powerful and resists the suppression that comes with growing up.

The **Parent** state reflects the absorption over the years of the influences of our actual parents and of parent and authority figures such as teachers, bosses and so on. It has two functions. One is to enable people to be better actual parents of their children. The other is to enable many responses to life to be made automatically—*that's the way it's done*—thereby freeing the Adult from making innumerable trivial decisions.

The Parent is like another internal language loop. It's a collection of pre-recorded, pre-judged, prejudiced codes for living. When a person is in the Parent ego state, they think, feel and behave like one of their parents or someone who took their place. The Parent decides, without reasoning, how to react to situations, what's good or bad, and how people should live. The Parent judges for or against and can be controlling or supportive. When the Parent is critical it's called the *Critical Parent*. When it's supportive, it's called the *Nurturing Parent*.

The **Adult** state is where we hope to be as adults. It's our adult selves, dealing with the vicissitudes of everyday life. It also has the function of regulating the activities of the Parent and Child, and mediating between them. When in the Adult state, the person functions as a human computer. It operates on data it collects and stores or uses to make decisions according to a logic-based programme. When in the Adult state, the person uses logical thinking to solve problems, making sure that Child or Parent emotions do not contaminate the process.

Eric Berne used this model of transactional analysis, which is the study of the transactions, the communication, and the *relationships* between people.

If you're communicating with someone and both of you are reasonable, logical and in a nice calm state, you'll both tend to communicate with each other from and to your Adult state, as below:

Effective Transactions

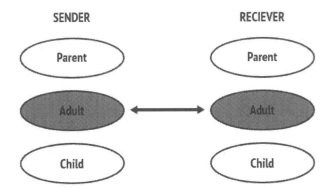

Since the Adult state is all about logic and rationality, we would ideally like to ensure that all communications in the workplace are Adult – Adult. After all, we're all supposed to act like adults in the workplace, and that should be the basis for the vast majority of our relationships there. In reality, though, it often doesn't work that way as there are times when these interactions become crossed.

Crossed Transactions

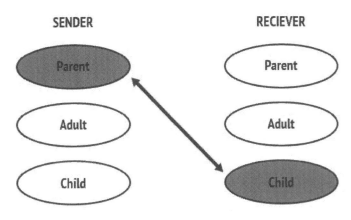

In a crossed transaction, the most frequently problematic issue is the Parent – Child communication. Here, the person initiating the conversation may feel stressed, or may habitually speak to others in a demeaning or bullying way, treating the other person as a child.

First, let's remind ourselves of a couple of key facts about this model:

- we possess all three states in our consciousness. Our personality is a result partly of our cumulative life experiences. Who we are as a Parent, Adult, or Child is a function of these experiences, no matter how we may wish to depart from them
- although we can learn new behaviours and skills, often what we *intend* in a transaction is not how the receiver interprets it
- all states are appropriate at some stage and in the right context. The challenge is to recognize what's appropriate and helpful.

In this crossed example above, where the Sender is speaking to the Receiver, it's coming across as a Parent – Child transaction which is one of the hardest to manage.

Sender as Parent:

- you may have had to follow-up several times about a recurring issue, so you're frustrated with the other person's performance. You're impatient and your disappointment is clear in your voice and body language

- you're anxious about getting a big assignment done and need the input of someone else. They may or may not be aware of the pressure you're under, but your tension comes across, including in your non-verbal behaviours
- you're very good at details and often have valuable insights, so you review things in detail and almost always have suggestions for everything others can do.

<u>Receiver as Child:</u>

- I'm trying here and I feel I have *disappointed* the authority figure (i.e. the boss).
- the person who's speaking to me sounds like my Dad or Mum when I was a teenager and came home late after curfew
- you may feel that the authority figures (such as the boss) feel don't trust you to perform adequately, even when you've been doing the work for some time.

The key here is to heighten our awareness of how our communication is being received. If we get into the Parent – Child mode too often with someone else, it can be frustrating and damaging to relationships.

Sadly, the pressures and stresses of life result in too many of us, too often inadvertently slipping into the Critical Parent state.

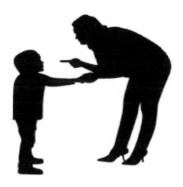

Public Domain Pictures[x]

When we do this, it's highly likely to trigger in the other person an Adapted Child response. Our challenge is twofold. First, to avoid using the Critical Parent mode with other adults, and secondly, if we do experience it from others, to manage our reactions in a way which keeps us where we ideally want to be, which is in Adult mode. A big challenge, for sure, and a lifetime's work!

The key factor here, again, is *awareness;* awareness of the pattern as it happens, and awareness of our response, followed by useful choices about how to avoid getting trapped in an unhelpful pattern.

The OK Corral

Another key factor is how, deep down, we feel about ourselves; and how, deep down, we feel about others. In his work, Eric Berne suggested that we are all born *OK,* i.e. we feel good about ourselves and about others. But then in 1971, a psychologist called Franklin Ernst, noticed that often, many of the problems in our relationships resulted from times when, for whatever reason, we take the view that we are not *OK* either with ourselves and/or with others. And so, Franklin Ernst developed the following model (in his *Handbook of Listening*) which is helpful in all kinds of contexts, not least when we need to engage in a difficult conversation. It's called the *OK Corral*:

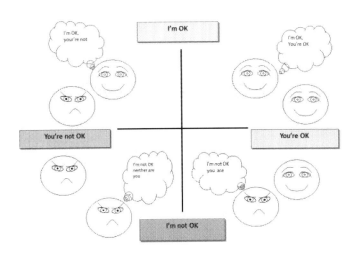

I'm not OK - You're OK

When I think I'm not OK but you are OK, then I'm putting myself in an inferior position with respect to you. This position may come from being belittled as a child, perhaps from dominant parents or maybe careless teachers or bullying peers.

I'm OK - You're not OK

People in this position feel themselves superior in some way to others, who are seen as inferior and not OK. As a result, they may be contemptuous and quick to anger. Their talk about others will be smug and supercilious, contrasting their own relative perfection with the limitation of others. Sadly, this position is a trap into which many managers, parents and others in authority may fall, assuming that their given position makes them better and, by implication, others are not OK.

I'm OK – You're OK

When I consider myself OK and also think of others as OK, then there is no position for me or you to be inferior or superior. This is, in many ways, the ideal position. Here, the person is comfortable with other people and with themself. They are confident, happy and get on with other people even when there are points of disagreement. Their relationships will be Adult to Adult.

I'm not OK – You're not OK

This is a relatively rare position, but perhaps occurs where people feel desperate. As a result, they remain feeling bad whilst also perceive others as bad.

Difficult Conversations

Clearly, when planning to have a difficult conversation, or even when having one, it's important to hold a strong positive belief in yourself (to feel OK about yourself), as well as having a strong positive belief in the other person (they're OK), i.e. to be operating in the top right hand quadrant.

But, in reality, we all know that in the heat of the moment, we can too easily find ourselves losing our patience and even our temper, raising our voice, and moving into a place where we find ourselves blaming the other person, i.e. into the bottom right hand quadrant of *I'm OK, You're not OK.*

Even if and when we succeed in developing such awareness, our interactions with others will always throw up new challenges. There will always be occasions when we need to have one of those difficult conversations. Tim Ferriss, an American entrepreneur and author once said:

> *A person's success in life can be measured by the number of uncomfortable conversations they are willing to have*

The need, from time to time, to have difficult conversations is pretty much a human universal. Many people are very good at avoiding them, both at work and at home in family life. And for those of us who do seek to have them, it takes enormous skill to stay in that Adult – Adult relationship we describe above.

Our experience of working with people over the years is that curiously, perhaps, many of us would prefer to bury our head in sand rather than have difficult (and important) conversations.

It seems more natural for us to be afraid of our own possible response, or of the response of others, if we do find ourselves in a difficult conversation. And yet, we all know that it rarely makes sense to say nothing, or to leave the "unsaid" unsaid, since this normally only makes things worse, storing up bigger problems into the future.

In the next section, therefore, we would like to provide a few valuable insights and tools about why this is so and what we can do about it which is better.

A difficult conversation is all about relationships: with ourselves and with others. So, in practice, here are some top tips to help us stay in the *I'm OK, You're OK* state of mind:

<u>Preparation</u>

For challenging or difficult topics, it's best to plan to have the conversation in advance: *I'd like to talk with you about...* or *We really need to talk about...* Then, mutually agree on a time and a place for the conversation and agree to meet in a place with enough space for all participants to be comfortable enough and to see each other clearly.

It's never helpful to collect and hold on to feelings of frustration, <u>anger</u>, or resentment for days, weeks, or longer, and then dump them on another person all at once. Whenever possible, try to discuss challenging issues as they come up or soon thereafter.

<u>Ground Rules</u>

- as much as possible, stay at about the same eye level. In other words, it's best if everyone participating is either seated or standing. It's generally not helpful for one person to be physically above or below others

- speak directly to the other person(s)
- speak as calmly in a matter-of-fact tone as possible. This maximizes the chances that others will hear the content of your message, rather than fixate on your emotions
- avoid finger-pointing, whether blaming or literally pointing fingers. This tends to make the other person(s) feel that he or she is being lectured or put down
- avoid name-calling, yelling, screaming, cursing, put-downs, insults, or threats (emotional or physical). When any of these happen, the only thing other people hear is anger and attack. As a result, they're likely to leave, shut down, or attack as well
- in describing your concerns and the things you'd like to happen differently, be as clear as possible and use specific examples. Avoid the words *always, never, everything*, and *nothing*. These may express frustration and upset, but they overgeneralize and are often fundamentally inaccurate
- no interrupting. When the other person is speaking, consciously *listen* to what he or she has to say with the intent of hearing it. This is very different from waiting for the other person to finish speaking so you can respond. If you're thinking about what you're going to say in response, while he or she is still speaking, you're probably not listening well

- make sure you understand what the other person has said before you respond. If you're not sure what he or she said or meant, ask for clarification. *Could you please repeat that?* Or *I'm not sure what you mean. Can you please help me better understand?*

- approach the conversation with <u>openness</u> and an interest in problem solving, rather than needing to be *right.* Anytime we see it as a competition where we need to be *right,* it means the other person has to be *wrong.* This kind of rigid either-or, win-lose, or right-wrong mindset makes conflict much more likely and mutual understanding much less likely

- keep to the topic at hand. Focus on the topic of this conversation. Bringing up issues or complaints related to other topics or past events always interferes with healthy communication during the current conversation. Save those other issues for another time. If they continue to be important to you, you'll remember them

- don't walk away or leave the conversation without the other person's agreement. Allow for the possibility of time-outs. It's important to discuss and mutually agree to the concept of a time-out as needed. Time-outs are not just for young children or professional sports teams. If things start to become too heated, it's important for people to be able to take a time-out. Time-outs give people the opportunity and the space to calm down and compose themselves, making it possible to continue

- take responsibility for feeling the way you do, rather than blaming the other person. No one can

make you feel a specific way. Use I statements —
as in, *I feel...* Be clear and specific about what the
other person did that contributed to your reaction.
Rather than saying, *You make me so mad,* focus on
the other person's actual behaviours

Finally, we leave you with another tip for difficult
conversations, which is a simple but powerful model with the
acronym of **CEDAR**:

C	Clarify	Say that you need to discuss something important with the other person and suggest that you both set aside a good time and place to discuss it. Possibly allow the other person time to think about
E	Explain	When the agreed time comes for the discussion, explain "why" the topic is important to discuss, and appreciate the other person for setting time aside to discuss it
D	Discuss	Listen to the other person's view; make sure your view is expressed and understood; and explore the pros and cons...possibly being open to new possibilities and options

A	Agree	Agree what you need to agree, and make sure both parties are clear about what's been agreed
R	Review	Agree when you will both review progress

Even though we now know all about the CEDAR model for difficult conversations, all about the OK Corral, and all about Eric Berne's work on the Adult, Parent and Child state, our action planning for change may still encounter other obstacles that could stop us from achieving our outcomes. Here's another, very valuable and even deeper insight into the inner world of the human being: the world of personal scripts – which can have a powerful hold on how we act and interact in the world.

Awareness of our own life story and script

As children, most of us loved story time and for many of us who still love reading books, watching the soaps on TV or going to see films or to the theatre, we still love the power of stories.

But often, there is a real story closer to home than in a book. It's our own personal story. But we're probably not even aware that we've written it. We began writing it from the day we were born and continued it throughout our childhood. By the time we were four we had the first draft version, then when we turned seven the entire story was pretty much complete.

From this point on we continued to refine and polish it throughout our adolescence, and often beyond into adulthood.

This story is otherwise known as our *life script*. The theory of life scripts was developed by Eric Berne in the 60s. According to Berne, each of us have a life script, although most of us are probably not aware of it. Our life scripts are created in childhood through the transactions between us as children and our parental influences. They partly programme our behaviour in later life. Often we are not aware of where they come from, or even that they exist at all.

These scripts have an unconscious effect on how we live our lives. They impact our decisions and influence what we believe we can achieve. They shape the image we have of ourselves. Depending on our particular script, we can interpret an event in a number of different ways. This is one of the reasons why two people can view the same event completely differently.

Whatever role we create for ourselves in our script, we can begin to perceive it as set in stone. We can even allow our script to shape the way we expect things to turn out in the future based on the role we are playing.

Life scripts primarily come from the messages (verbal and non verbal) given to us in our earliest childhood by our parents and other key influences. As tiny babies and young children, our brains pay a lot attention to:

- observing how others behave
- what we're told as a child that we must be; and what's expected or wanted of us. This can come in the form of labelling. *You're just like X relative or You're... clever, naughty, the best, clumsy, strong, different, awful etc*
- the demands from our parents in our childhood aimed at stopping us from doing something

All of these things inform the life scripts we create in our childhood, and which we can then take with us into adulthood.

Common Life Scripts:

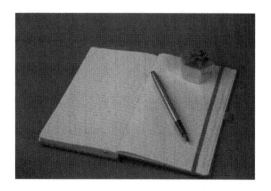

Do any of these sounds familiar to you?

- Everyone else is better than me
- I'm unlucky, bad things always happen to me

- I'm a loser
- I'm always the victim in situations
- I can't make friends easily
- I'm terrible at learning languages, I can never pick them up
- I'm too fat and can't lose weight, I won't be content until I'm slimmer
- I'm unlucky in love, I never meet the right person
- People always leave me
- I won't be happy until I meet someone
- I'm not good enough
- I can't do it on my own

These are all examples of life scripts and sometimes it's these life scripts that get in the way and stop us from achieving happiness. There are positive scripts of course which can be empowering, but it's the negative ones which can severely limit our lives if we let them shape our future behaviour. We can start to believe them and let them define us and how we live our lives. If history always seems to be repeating itself, maybe it's because the same script is playing over and over. So what can we do? Sometimes as we've said before, recognising we have a negative life script is the first key step to shift it.

Researcher Mel Johnson (www.bestselfology.com/life-scripts/) has developed Eric Berne's work to suggest that these patterns, if allowed to play out in our lives, can result in some of the following life scripts:

People always leave me

Could this be you?

- you wait for invitations rather than invite people to events, as proof of your popularity
- you get jealous very easily, and invent reasons for arguments, to test people's love

I always put other people first

Could this be you?

- you go out of your way to do favours for other people
- you feel that you're more generous than the people around you

I'm not good enough

Could this be you?

- you self-sabotage, creating excuses for your anticipated failure
- you avoid competitive situations – even playing board games or sports – because you fear coming last

I can't do it on my own

Could this be you?

- you're attracted to people who you see as being stronger than you are
- you're the first to admit that you lack common sense, or that you're hopeless around the house

Bad things happen to me more than they do to other people

Could this be you?

- you find it easy to imagine the worst possible outcome
- you have regularly been accused of being overly cautious and protective

I deserve this

Could this be you?

- you feel that other people don't recognise your talents or abilities
- you suspect that others are holding you back

What can we do with this information about life scripts? Of course, the very first thing to do is seek to surface what script might be driving some or all of our approach to life. Once we are aware of the potential operation of a life script, we can begin to exercise more choice in our lives, and possibly take action which goes off script if that is a useful thing to do.

Our life script is individual to each of us. To uncover it, it's necessary to identify the patterns in our life, particularly if we feel that they can be destructive.

Here's a powerful exercise which we can each use to surface the script that may unconsciously be driving some or much of our approach to life. It's called *Once upon a Time.*

Find yourself in a calm state, and give yourself thirty minutes or so of private, uninterrupted space, equipped with a pen and paper or a keyboard. Write down these words:

Once upon a time, there was a boy/girl called [add your name here] who was born in [insert year]….

And then write down the first things that come to your mind about your life, starting from your early childhood and ***as if you're describing the life of someone else…***

Then, maybe, if you wish, put the story away for a day or two. When you're ready, review your story and look for any patterns you see… helpful or unhelpful.

And then, of course, explore whether and to what extent you want to have more choice in your life, and set outcomes appropriately, using the life planning and outcomes section described in this book in chapters three and four.

Here's a summary of the *Once Upon a Time* exercise:

Step	
1	Find yourself in a calm state, and give yourself 30 minutes or so of private, uninterrupted space, equipped with a pen and paper or a keyboard. Write down these words: ***Once upon a time, there was a [boy/girl] called [add your name], who was born in [add your year of birth]……..***"
2	Write a page or two of the first years of your life, as if you were writing about someone else. Always refer to yourself as *he* or *she*. Write whatever comes to mind
3	Leave this document for a while: preferably look at it again the following day
4	When you review the document, look for any recurring patterns of thought, feelings or actions that began in your early years and which still show up in your life
5	Review the pros and con of such patterns; and explore which patterns, if any, are helpful; and which, if any, are destructive and which you want to get rid of

6	Think about any new patterns that you would most like to build into your life, using some of the relevant tools and techniques in this book, leading you into clear new goals and outcomes

It's not uncommon for people to ask themselves fundamental questions about the meaning and direction of their lives at certain points in their life, such as for example, in their mid-thirties (midlife), when people may often want to take stock and re-evaluate. For this reason, we're now about to move onto the different stages of our life journey.

Stages of our life journey

Just as a book is split into chapters, and plays are split into acts, so our lives take on their own shape, as we move from childhood to adulthood. But this simple two-way categorisation does not really do justice to the rich series of stages we go through from birth to death.

Most of us have probably heard the term *midlife* or even *midlife* crisis so maybe such terms give us a better flavour of the natural transitions we all find ourselves going through.

Thomas Armstrong's research (2007) points to the following stages of life and their very best aspects:

Age	Stage of Life and its Best Aspects
0 -3 yrs	**Infancy** Full of vitality and boundless energy
3 – 6 yrs	**Early childhood** Full of playfulness, curiousity and inventiveness
6 – 8 yrs	**Middle childhood** Characterised by lots of imagination, as the child's inner, subjective sense starts to develop
8 – 11 yrs	**Late childhood** More and more use of inventive solutions to solve pratical problems: ingenuity
11 – 20 yrs	**Adolescence** Development of emotional, social and sexual awareness. Potential development and awareness of how the self can differ from others

20 – 35 yrs	**Early adulthood** Importance of establishing a personal life, possibly free from others in the close family, of finding a home, a partner, a job, a distinct identity and standing on one's own feet
35 – 50 yrs	**Midlife** A stage of life often characterised by reflection on the deeper meaning of life; contemplation on whether what the peson has got, is what they really want; taking stock and possibly considering other options
50 – 80 yrs	**Mature adulthood** The beginning of sharing of expertise and wisdom to the next generation
80 yrs +	**Late adulthood** A stage of life characterised by insight, wisdom, generosity of spirit to help the younger generations; and actions to secure a positive legacy

As Thomas Armstrong writes:

Since each stage of life has its own unique gift to give to humanity, we need to do whatever we can to support each stage, and to protect each stage from attempts to suppress its individual contribution to the human life cycle. Thus, we need to be wary, for example, of attempts to thwart a young child's need to play through the establishment high-pressure formal academic preschools. We should protect the wisdom of aged from elder abuse. We need to do what we can to help our adolescents at risk. We need to advocate for prenatal education and services for poor mothers, and support safe and healthy birthing methods in third world countries. We ought to take the same attitude toward nurturing the human life cycle as we do toward saving the environment from global warming and industrial pollutants. For by supporting each stage of the human life cycle, we will help to ensure that all of its members are given care and helped to blossom to their fullest degree

And of course, we humans have instinctively known for centuries that each life stage brings its own special gifts and challenges:

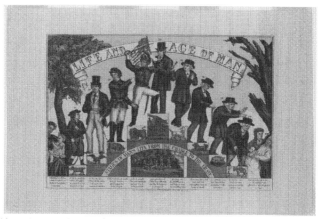

Life and Age of Man; Stages of Man's Life from the cradle to the grave
(Lithograph, 1856-1907)
Library of Congress[xi]

William Shakespeare too was aware of similar stages of life when he wrote the speech about *The Seven Ages of Man* in his play *As You Like It:*

> *They have their exits and entrances;*
> *And one man in his time plays many parts,*
> *His Acts being seven ages. At first the Infant,*
> *Mewling and puking in the nurse's arms.*
> *Then the whining Schoolboy, with his satchel*
> *And shining morning face, creeping like snail*
> *Unwillingly to school. And then the Lover,*
> *Sighing like furnace, with a woeful ballad*
> *Made to his mistress' eyebrow. Then a Soldier,*
> *Full of strange oaths, and bearded like the pard;*
> *Jealous in honour, sudden and quick in quarrel,*
> *Seeking the bubble reputation,*
> *Even in the cannon's mouth. And then the Justice,*
> *In fair round belly with good capon lined,*
> *With eyes severe, and beard of formal cut,*

Full of wise saws and modern instances -
And so he plays his part. The sixth age shifts
Into the lean and slippered Pantaloon
With spectacles on nose, and pouch on side,
His youthful hose, well saved, a world too wide,
For his shrunk shank; and his big manly voice,
Turning again toward childish treble, pipes
And whistles in his sound. Last scene of all,
That ends this strange eventful history,
Is second childishness, and mere oblivion,
Sans teeth, sans eyes, sans taste, sans everything.

(William Shakespeare, 1599)

We conclude this chapter by sharing with you another important building block which can go a long way to help explain why some people seem more ready for change than other people, and at particular stages of their life. The model goes back as far as 1943 and has withstood well the test of time. It's the work of Abraham Maslow, and his *Hierarchy of Human Needs* model.

Maslow's Hierarchy of Needs Model

In his influential paper of 1943, *A Theory of Human Motivation,* psychologist Abraham Maslow proposed that healthy human beings have a certain number of needs, and that these needs are arranged in a hierarchy, with some needs (such as physiological and safety needs) being more primitive or basic than others (such as social and ego needs). Maslow's so-called *Hierarchy of Human Needs* model is often presented as a five-level pyramid, with higher needs coming into focus only once lower, more basic needs are met.

Maslow called the bottom four levels of the pyramid *deficiency needs* because a person does not feel anything if they are met, but becomes anxious if they are not. Thus, physiological needs such as eating, drinking, and sleeping are deficiency needs, as are safety needs, social needs such as friendship and sexual intimacy, and ego needs such as self-esteem and recognition. In contrast, Maslow called the fifth level of the pyramid a *growth need* because it enables a person to *self-actualize* or reach their fullest potential as a human being. Once a person has met their deficiency needs, they can turn their attention to self-actualization.

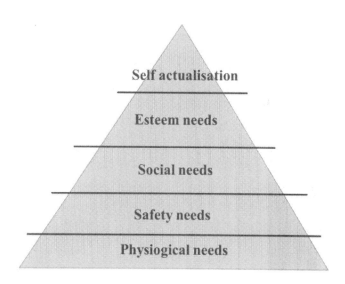

As we suggest above, the term midlife or midlife crisis is well recognised in our culture. When, possibly at the age of thirty-five or more, having worked hard to get some of our basic needs such as a good place to live, a close relationship and family, and a secure income, a person can wake up one morning and find themselves asking questions such as:

There must be more to life than this, but what is it?

Or they find they're in a job or occupation that bores them, and they need to find a role in life which brings more meaning. This is Armstrong's Life Stage Midlife (35 – 50 years), or possibly for some people occurs at a later stage, such as retirement.

A key part of happiness is being aware of these life stages and the special needs that some of them may bring, plus the tools and knowledge to enable you to meet these needs. For anyone who finds themselves asking the fundamental questions of life purpose and meaning, there are tools elsewhere in this book, such as the *Ikigai* tool explained in chapter one.

Someone calculated recently that if we live for eighty-five years, we have 31,025 days of life on the planet. It can do no harm every now and again to stop, pause and reflect on where we are on our life journey and do all we can to learn from the past and hope for the very best from the remaining days we hope to have.

We've covered a lot of territory in the book so far about some of the factors which govern our and others' happiness. The good news is that recent and extensive research has shown that all these factors are in fact different aspects of one important concept: *emotional intelligence.*

Emotional Intelligence

There used to be a time when the word *intelligence* meant just one thing, which was how *clever* or *brainy* a person is. Being brainy is helpful, especially if you're trying to solve a complex mathematical problem. There is, however, another type of intelligence. In 1993, Peter Salovey and John Mayer, researchers at Yale University coined the term *emotional intelligence*. They described emotional intelligence as:

The ability to monitor one's own and others' feelings and emotions, and to use this information to guide one's thinking and action

Since that time, the concept of emotional intelligence has been extensively researched, and is a critical factor in our personal, family and work lives.

Emotional intelligence involves all the issues we've explored so far in this book:

- how we manage our thoughts, our feelings and adjust our actions
- our self awareness and awareness of others and
- how we manage our relationships

These are all things that have a big bearing on our happiness and contribute (or not) to others' happiness.

At the heart of emotional intelligence is the connection between:

- what we think
- how we feel
- how we act

We saw this in chapter seven, in the following diagram:

Mind and Body Connection

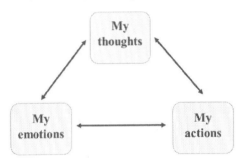

For example, if we think of sucking a lemon, we may feel our mouths go funny. If we start thinking about our favourite food, we can find our mouths salivating.

In chapter seven, we described the Triune Brain, and how the ancient lizard brain is thousands of times faster and stronger than our human brain. Unless we're self aware and careful, we can find ourselves in situations where our reactions, driven by our ancient lizard brain can completely take over and lead us to feel so angry and do stupid things which we later regret. Emotional intelligence gives us the skills to deal better with such situations, so that we manage our thinking and our emotions, and thus take the right actions instead.

We're fortunate now to have access to research which helps us understand how emotional intelligence works. Here's an example:

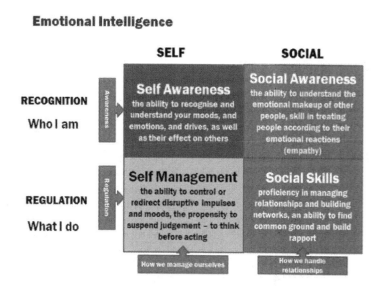

We can explore some scenarios and see which aspects of emotional intelligence are (or aren't) in play. (Suggested answers are in the Appendix).

Scenario 1

Someone you work with has grown up in a family where their every wish has been indulged and where there was no discipline. One day, they turn up at work in a foul mood and shout at people.

Which part or parts of the emotional intelligence model are low and creating this problem? If you were their boss, what would be the best thing to do to defuse the problem and help the person improve their performance?

Scenario 2

Someone in your family displays behaviours associated with a bully. They are driven to achieve great things in their life, and have high expectations of themselves – and others. They believe there is just *their way or the highway*. This results sometimes in open conflict with others, or in a hostile and fearful atmosphere in the family where people don't say what they really feel.

Which part or parts of the emotional intelligence model are low and creating this problem? As an adult in the family, what's the best thing to do to defuse the problem and help the person improve their performance?

Scenario 3

One of your relatives is very popular in your family because they're so keen to help everyone else. They're always first to offer help and support to other family members and to neighbours, for example by offering to do their shopping. They're exceptional at anticipating other people's needs. The trouble is that this person gets worn out, and every four – six weeks, feels so exhausted they take time off work, retreat to their bed for a week or so to recuperate. They're exasperated with this pattern, and have asked for your advice.

Which part or parts of the emotional intelligence model are in play here? As a concerned and caring adult in the family, what's the best thing you could do to help this person deal with the underlying issue(s)?

In the work context, the research of Maddocks and Hughes (2019) shows there are five key factors that contribute to emotional intelligence:

- paying attention to how others are feeling
- consulting and involving others where necessary
- investing time and energy in building relationships
- valuing individuals and respecting their views and opinions
- having faith in people whilst being realistic in expectations

We would suggest that these five factors are the essential ingredients for happiness whether at home, with family, with friends, in communities and organisations.

The good news is that our emotional intelligence skills are not set down in stone when we're born. These skills are used and practised each moment in our lives, including when we're quietly sitting alone and thinking, as well as when we're interacting with others.

All the tools and techniques described so far in this book support the development of emotional intelligence. For example:

- knowing our purpose, showing compassion and gratitude (chapter one)
- random acts of kindness (chapter one)
- self awareness and awareness of others (chapter two)
- seeing things from different perspectives (chapter two)
- practising mindfulness (chapter two)
- taking actions using the well-formed outcome model (chapter five)
- managing obstacles (chapter six)
- understanding how our brains work (chapter seven)
- managing our self-talk (chapter seven)
- enhancing our communication skills (chapter eight)
- patterns of thinking (chapter nine)
- understanding personality and relationships (chapter ten)

There are so many possible actions we can all take in response to reading this book, but there's one in particular which to us at least stands out in its potential to make the world a better place. This is the simple but powerful commitment to do *a random act of kindness* each day.

Finally on the topic of emotional intelligence, if you'd like more information and might even like to take an online assessment of your current emotional intelligence strengths and possible areas of development, here's a link to an excellent source of such information:

https://www.psionline.com/en-gb/emotional-intelligence

Much of this chapter has focussed on our relationships with ourselves and with others. In the big scheme of things, there's an even more important relationship we all have – our relationship with the planet that we live on. This relationship in turn is largely driven by the shared mindset we share about the world and how it works. This is where we're going next, our eighth Tool in the Happiness Toolkit. There's a common saying that *we can't see what's under our nose,* and this last tool is about uncovering some of the main assumptions that drive mankind's behaviours in relation to how we treat the planet; and questioning them. If we think our *shared mindsets* need to be updated/revised to create the new and better post Covid-19 normal and to create more happiness on the planet, let's do it!

Chapter eleven: Shared mindsets

The earlier chapters in this book have all dealt with how we can increase our own personal happiness, as well as other people's happiness. We now focus on a final and equally, (possibly more?) important issue, which is about how we can achieve happiness for ourselves and others without having an adverse effect on the planet. In chapter five, we introduced a tool (called *PESEO*) to help people check out whether any actions they intended to take fitted with their values and beliefs, i.e. the *ecology check*. So, in this chapter, we explore this additional and important dimension of happiness: how we can be happy without causing damage to nature and the world and how we might even be able to do some good, where we can.

In the Introduction, we suggested there are three nested circles that we need to explore and understand more of, in order to enhance our happiness. So, now, it's time to explore the outer circle: the consequences of our actions on the world.

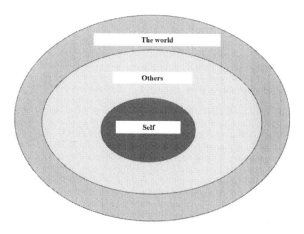

Let's start by reminding ourselves of the intention held by the Action for Happiness movement, which is:

> *We want to see a fundamentally different way of life – where people care less about what they can get for themselves and more about the happiness of others*

Now that we've begun to experience Covid-19, its impact on the world – and the human response to it (so far), what would *a fundamentally different way of life* be like? And how can we make the lifestyle associated with the *new normal* be good for our own personal happiness, others' happiness and the happiness of the planet? We've already seen some wonderful signs of how well and quickly nature can sometimes respond to reductions in human activity and these have been well documented in the news. Paradoxically, reductions in air pollution in certain parts of the world may have saved thousands of lives. According to Stanford University scientist

Marshall Burke, the reduction in air pollution may have helped save the lives of 77,000 people in China under the age of five, and over seventy years.

> *Given the huge amount of evidence that breathing dirty air contributes heavily to premature mortality, a natural – if admittedly strange – question is whether the lives saved from this reduction in pollution caused by economic disruption from Covid-19 exceed the death toll from the virus itself*
> (G-FEED science blog)

In the human domain too, there have been positive developments since the initial lockdown began; in certain places, more community spirit, more volunteering, more people walking out in nature, and more mindfulness. Equally, though, it's important to note that things in the human domain have not all been good. For example, a huge increase in domestic violence, emotional stress, unemployment, increases in anxiety and financial hardship.

One major theme from the initial lockdown period was the growing recognition of the important role that contact with nature makes to human happiness. Given the importance that nature plays in human happiness, we might well ask ourselves why so much we've achieved and enjoyed has been at the expense of the natural world. Inger Anderson, the UN's environment chief raised exactly this question in March 2020, when she said:

> *Nature is sending us a message that if we neglect the planet, we put our own wellbeing (and therefore happiness) at risk. Never before have so many opportunities existed for pathogens to pass from wild and domestic animals to people.*
>
> *Our continued erosion of wild spaces has brought us uncomfortably close to animals and plants that harbour diseases that can jump to humans.*
>
> *There are too many pressures at the same time on our natural systems and something has to give. We are intimately interconnected with nature, whether we like it or not. If we don't take care of nature, we can't take care of ourselves. And as we hurtle towards a population of 10 billion people on this planet, we need to go into this future armed with nature as our strongest ally*
>
> (Inger Anderson, in the Guardian on 25 March 2020)

As the Archbishop of Canterbury Justin Welby said in his Easter 2020 Sunday sermon, there should be the possibility of a better and happier world after the Covid-19 pandemic.

There's also now the well known graffiti in Hong Kong which appeared on a wall there in April 2020:

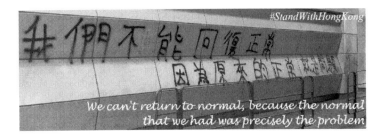

What needs to happen to create this *new and better normal* and what is our role in this? Certainly, a lot needs to change in our external world.

But as Robert Pirsig says in *Zen and the Art of Motorcycle Maintenance:*

> **If a factory is torn down but the thinking which produced it is left standing, then that way of thinking will simply produce another factory. If a revolution destroys a government, but the same kind of thinking that produced the government is left intact, then all future governments will repeat their mistakes**

In other words, there will need to be significant shifts in how we see and understand the world and our place in it, our **shared mindsets**, if you like. What we mean by this term is:

Definition of *shared mindsets*

> *The collection of quite deeply embedded beliefs, commonly shared in our society, about how human beings relate to the world; how human beings relate to and treat the natural world; how our economies should operate; and how our society should be structured*

This takes us straight to the final and eighth Tool in our Happiness Toolkit:

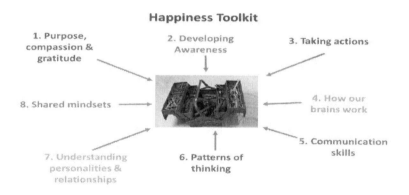

Happiness Toolkit

1. Purpose, compassion & gratitude

2. Developing Awareness

3. Taking actions

8. Shared mindsets

4. How our brains work

7. Understanding personalities & relationships

6. Patterns of thinking

5. Communication skills

Here's an interesting question. How would you define the dominant Western world shared mindset?

There's no single correct answer to this question, and not everyone would agree, (but in this context that's okay). To attempt to answer this question, we've looked back at the broad shape of society over the last few centuries. For us, themes that emerge include:

- individual effort should be rewarded more than collective effort
- all natural resources are there to be used and exploited
- profit is good, regardless of how it is achieved
- perpetual growth in all economies in the world is good
- external manifestations of wealth are more important than acts of kindness or charity

Our shared mindset about how we should relate to nature is particularly important since, as we've recognised above, we now more than ever value the role that nature plays in our happiness.

How is it that our society has such a dismissive view of the natural world? Here's a suggestion that not everyone may agree with, but we believe it's worth considering. About 3,000 years ago, in the Old Testament, Moses wrote:

We are to have dominion over the fish of the sea, and over the birds of the air, and over the cattle, and over all the wild animals of the earth, and over every creeping thing that creeps upon the earth (Gen 1:26)

About 3,000 years ago, when there were only a few thousand humans in the Middle East, it may well have been appropriate to have such a view of the relationship between humans and nature; but now in 2020, when there will soon be more than 7 billion humans on the planet, many of whom have unprecedented expectations of consumption, we would suggest it's time for us humans to develop a more constructive relationship with nature and build this into our mainstream Western mindset.

There's another aspect of Western culture that needs exploring. It's the tendency to assume that the problems and challenges we face are mostly independent of each other. For example, in the medical world, many people go to see the doctor to resolve a problem such as a bad back and come away happy with a prescription for some new pills. But research in Canada, by the Ontario Healthy Communities Commission, clearly shows how our health and well-being are affected by a multitude of other factors:

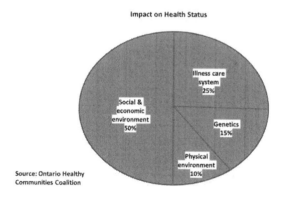

Impact on Health Status

Illness care system 25%

Social & economic environment 50%

Genetics 15%

Physical environment 10%

Source: Ontario Healthy Communities Coalition

Fortunately, there are lots of enlightened folk in the NHS who do understand that many factors interact with each other to shape our personal health and well-being. There's now a significant movement in the NHS which means that sometimes a GP will recognise that the best solution might not be another pill, but a different course of action entirely. This is sometimes called social prescribing.

In mainstream Western culture, we've been taught to analyse, to use our rational ability to trace paths from cause and effect, to look at things in small and understandable pieces, and to solve problems by seeking to control the world, as if we have *dominion* over it.

On the other hand, there are alternative mindsets to this. For example, in some Eastern traditions, particularly Buddhist cultures, there's a mindset which regards the sanctity of all living creatures; which understands that humans are just part of nature, not dominating it; and which sees the whole as greater than the sum of the parts.

A helpful summary of some of the key Buddhist teachings can be found at:

https://www.bbc.co.uk/bitesize/guides/z4b42hv/revision/3

In the last few years, there's been a growing number of people in the West who are clear that there need to be changes to the traditional Western mindset, most notably perhaps the Transition Movement, the various Green parties in different countries, and Extinction Rebellion. And in addition, there's been a growing interest first kickstarted in 1990 by Peter Senge from the MIT Sloane School of Management, with his book, *The Fifth Discipline*. As a result of his pioneering thinking, there's now a strong movement called "systems thinking", which has at its core the insight that in the world, everything is connected to everything else, and it's the relationships and interconnections between things and people that are most important.

Systems thinking draws some of its lessons from nature, recognising that in the natural world, everything is connected to everything else. A good metaphor here is the spider's web:

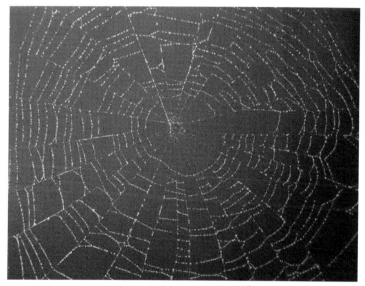

Photo courtesy Steve Gibson[xii]

A spider's web is constructed so that if any part of it is disturbed, a reaction is felt across the entire web, alerting the spider to its trapped and struggling insect food.

In addition, it's constructed so that failure in one area will not cause the entire web to fail but will forfeit only the failing section.

As John Muir (an influential American naturalist and author) once wrote:

When we try to pick out anything by itself,
we find it hitched to everything else in the
universe

A system is a set of interrelated elements that make a unified whole. Individual things—like plants, people, schools, watersheds, or economies—are themselves systems and at the same time cannot be fully understood apart from the larger systems in which they exist. It's quite useful to see all our lives as a complex web of inter-related connections, where a single change in one part of the web can affect other parts of the web. During the Covid-19 initial lockdown, we each saw how our lives are so intimately affected by other parts of the web:

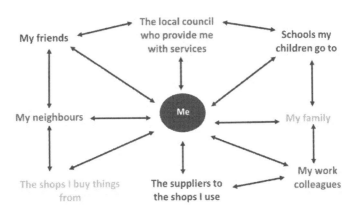

Systems thinking accepts that our lives are intimately interconnected with everything else. A systems lens helps people to understand the complexity of the world around us, and encourages us think about relationships, and connectedness.

As we all observe the responses of world leaders to Covid-19, we don't see any clear vision at all that if and when *normal* reappears, it will be any different from the old normal, i.e. can we rely on traditional, old thinking and behaviours to get back to normal? If we want a new and better normal, we need to stop doing something old: and that something surely must be to revise the mainstream Western shared mindset to some degree.

As Sir David Attenborough wrote:

> ***Think this world is precious, think your time is precious, think the rest of the natural world is precious and all those things need cherishing – that's the fundamental attitude. The world is not a bowl of fruit from which we can just take what we wish. We are part of it, and if we destroy it, we destroy ourselves***
>
> (Sir David Attenborough, in the Independent Newspaper, 19 April 2020)

We all have a choice: do we sit back and wait for everyone else to recognise that something needs to change about our normal shared mindset, or do we take action ourselves to create our own new mindset and then watch with delight as we see others do the same thing? The best way to predict our future is to create it.

Given that we want greater happiness for ourselves and our loved ones, how do we ensure this does not come at the expense of the world? How do we go about adopting a different shared mindset which is likely to result in a new and better normal, and thus increase happiness in ourselves, others and on the planet?

The good news is that by committing to take actions from earlier parts of this book, you're already taking advantage of this more interconnected way of thinking. All the tools and techniques in this book are based on the premise that if we take a tiny action in one part of our life, there're bound to be changes in other parts of our world, i.e. as we say in chapter seven, a change in our thoughts is likely to create a change in our feelings and possibly through into our actions.

We conclude this book by referring you to another of the very best thinkers and writers on leadership, and this is Professor Dan Goleman from Harvard University, who is prominent in the field of emotional intelligence. He has co-written a book called *Ecoliterate*, in which he pleas for us to develop a new mindset based more on at least three factors:

- developing empathy for all forms of life
- making the invisible visible
- anticipating unintended consequences

Let's take each of these in turn:

<u>Developing empathy for all forms of life</u>

We've already seen that in our traditional Western mindset there's a belief that we're somehow separate from and superior to the rest of nature, making it okay for us to exploit, degrade and pollute the planet.

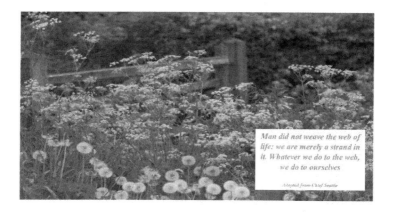

Man did not weave the web of life: we are merely a strand in it. Whatever we do to the web, we do to ourselves

Adapted from Chief Seattle

The number of humans on the planet currently increases by about 83 million per year. If we go back to 1800, there were only 1 billion of us. Right now, there are 7.7 billion humans on the planet. Current estimates are that, unless something exceptional happens, by the mid 2030s there will be 9 billion and by the mid 2050s, the figure will be 10 billion.

In terms of technology and with our dominant mindset, we're so powerful, so all pervasive, the mechanisms we have for destruction are so wholesale and so frightening that we can exterminate whole ecosystems without even noticing it. We already know that, for example, the plastics problem in the seas is wreaking appalling damage to marine life. Now the human species can go everywhere: we can go to the bottom of the sea, we can go into space, we can use drones, we can use helicopters. We can use intrude, invade and pollute almost every aspect of the living world.

One of the finest thinkers about life was the English anthropologist, Gregory Bateson, who in 1972 very clearly analysed the issue thus:

The major problems in the world are the result of the difference between how nature works and the way people think

That's why, in a nutshell, we need as a species to develop a new and different shared mindset about the world, and one which includes much more empathy with the natural world.

Dan Goleman, in conjunction with the Center for Ecology (www.ecoliteracy.org), suggests we need to shift this part of our mindset in a way which recognises humans as being part of the web of life. This reinforces the view of the UN's environment chief, Inger Andersen, that:

Nature is sending us a message that if we neglect the planet, we put our own wellbeing (and therefore happiness) at risk

There are lots of tiny, but significant ways we could each choose to take action here, including: being more mindful of nature (for more on mindfulness, see chapter two): or doing what we can to promote the natural world around us, whether it be our garden, our patio or balcony. If you're interested in increasing biodiversity by encouraging, for example, more butterflies into your garden, there's an excellent book on this by Jane Moore, *Planting for Butterflies* (2020).

Making the invisible visible

When we buy something, it will have come from somewhere, been grown or manufactured, and will have been transported from somewhere to the shop where we buy it. Some workers will have worked hard to get it to us, in good condition and on time and they'll be subject to certain (often poor) working conditions. In Stroud High Street, in the UK, there's a shop called the *Art of Clay*, (run by an artist called Clay), which has a sign outside that reads:

Every pound you spend is a vote for the world you want to live in

As consumers, the more we can become aware of and critically ask questions about our consumption, the easier it will be to make the invisible consequences of our consumption visible. For example, if we know the nice, fresh food produce we're buying is flown in from a country which still struggles to feed its own people, would we still want to buy it? If we know that the nice cheap clothing we want to buy is made by people in a country thousands of miles away who have to work as virtual modern day slaves – would we still choose to buy it?

There's already some evidence that one of the consequences of the pandemic may be a shift in some of our buying habits. According to Barclaycard, spending at local shops rose by almost forty percent in April 2020. Of course, this behaviour may have been influenced by other factors such as long queues elsewhere, but a separate survey by the same card provider found that many people were planning to increase their spending at local butchers, cafes and farmers' markets in the future.

At least, the easiest thing we can do is to step back, pause occasionally and ask ourselves questions about where and how we use our purchasing power. For as Anthony Robbins (2001) writes:

The quality of our lives is a direct
reflection of the quality of the
questions we ask ourselves

<u>Anticipating unintended consequences</u>

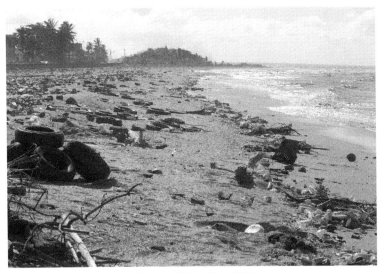

photo by Nilys Ally, 2010

With this alternative mindset, where we recognise that lots of things are connected with other things, the law of unintended consequences explains how, when one simple change is made to a part of a situation, we can inadvertently cause unintended consequences in other things.

The concept of unintended consequences can be attributed to Adam Smith, the Scottish economist and philosopher who in 1776 wrote *The Wealth of Nations*. He used the term the *invisible hand* to describe the unintended consequences of certain economic activity. The image above shows a clear example of unintended consequences: when we buy something made of plastic, none of us intends that it will end up polluting the ocean or getting washed on a beach thousands of miles away. Unintended consequences can also be positive, for example, one of the unintended consequences of the UK's response to Covid-19 and the initial lockdown policy was to create in at least some communities a stronger self-help culture and more community resilience. But, equally, we have to bear in mind there were severe negative unintended consequences such as more poverty, more suicides and more domestic violence.

In the new and better normal world we all seek, the more we can anticipate possible unintended consequences, the better; seeking to reduce the negative ones whilst encouraging the positive ones.

Changing our mindset about how the world works, and how we should best interact with the world is not easily done and certainly not done overnight. One is reminded of that rather strange saying: *How do you eat an elephant: one bite at a time.* In other words, decide on one small step, and take it.

For example, here's a possible action to consider:

With everything I buy, I'll think about whether it's the best choice for me, bearing in mind what I can find out about its environmental cost to the planet, as well as its financial cost to me

And then, to use the amazing ability of the brain to create habits, by reviewing our success and make whatever we choose to do an embedded habit.

As John Seymour and Joseph O'Connor (1990) say:

If we want to change the world, we must first change ourselves

Actions and habits of this sort are guaranteed to make us happier, others happier and the planet happier. And guess what? By taking such action, we'll not be alone – others will be taking similar actions and together, we can create a positive and widespread ripple effect, changing the way we humans live on the planet.

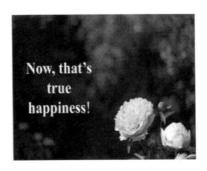

Epilogue

In this book, we've explored eight Tools in the Happiness Toolkit, and there are certainly even more aspects of happiness than this. And with each tool, there is so much ground to cover. In this context, it might be tempting to simply give up, shrug one's shoulders, and walk away from taking any actions to promote happiness in oneself or with others. Of course, chapter three gives some pointers about *Where to Start*.

Covid-19 has shown us that when humanity is united in a common cause, rapid change is possible. None of the world's problems are technically difficult to solve; they often occur when humans disagree. On the other hand, when our societies are at their best, humanity's creative powers are boundless. A few months ago, the vastly increased use of cycle tracks and walkways in city centres would have seemed impossible, so too some of the more radical changes we're making in our social behaviour, economy and the role of government in our lives.

The questions for us to answer now are what do we want to achieve and what kind of world do we want to create? When the initial crisis subsides, we might even ask whether we want to return to *normal* or whether there might be a *new and better normal?* We might ask what parts of the economy and society will we want to restore, and what parts might we choose to let go. The threat of further waves or new infectious diseases remains. Our response today can set a course for the future.

People are asking questions that have until now lurked on activist margins. How do we create a fairer world to protect and support those who are vulnerable and at the same time steward the resources of our planet so it can be handed on to the next generation?

What was so beguiling about the Western lifestyle that came to an abrupt end in March 2020? Or was it a case of Hans Christian Andersen's story of *The Emperor's New Clothes* with no-one daring to say they didn't like the constant rush, the desperate need to fill each and every moment of the day and night, the obsession with the cult of celebrity and the consumer frenzy for fear of appearing weird, a loser, a Billy no Mates? For a very long time now, (probably hundreds of years but especially in the last thirty years or so), human societies have focussed more on *external wealth,* acquiring ever brighter, better and more on trend stuff, on *doing* rather than *being.*

As Covid-19 stirs our compassion, more and more of us realize that we don't want to go back to a normal so sorely lacking it. We have the opportunity now to forge a new, more compassionate normal. But there is an equally long tradition in human culture of *internal wealth* i.e. how to be a good human being, how to have great relationships with other humans and with the planet.

In this book, it's been our aim to bring together some of the best insights, tools and techniques about how to live a great life and how to be happy. Interestingly, Yale University is running a free online course called *The Science of Wellbeing* which covers some of the material explored in this book. Nearly 3 million people have registered for this course, and this is another valuable way of continuing our personal development, if we so choose. The link to this course is:

https://www.coursera.org/learn/the-science-of-well-being

Let's make more use of all this wisdom to create a new and better normal where our happiness is not created to the detriment of other people and the planet on which we all depend.

We have a Facebook page where people can, if they wish, share and explore any of the issues raised in this book and the *new and better normal* so many of us now seek. It can be found at:

https://www.facebook.com/Finding-Happiness-after-Covid-19-103335108060770

Appendix

Answers to the Quiz (chapter nine) on the Emergenetics
Thinking Styles

	Statement	Which Thinking Style is this?
1	What are the facts here?	Analytical style
2	How do other people feel about this?	Social style
3	What are the next steps?	Structural style
4	Imagine how this could change the future	Conceptual style
5	I need to ask how this fits with our values	Social style
6	How practical is all this?	Structural style
7	I wonder what new opportunities this creates for us?	Conceptual style
8	Logically, this makes no sense	Analytical style
9	What's the missing information here?	Analytical style

10	What's the correct procedure for this?	Structural style
11	What would others expect from us?	Social style
12	Just imagine the new options this opens up..	Conceptual style

Suggested answers to the three scenarios in chapter ten on emotional intelligence

Emotional Intelligence

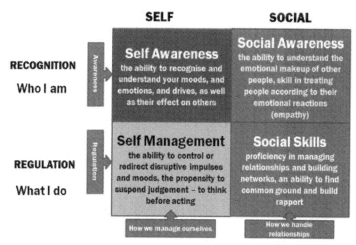

Scenario 1

Someone you work with has grown up in a family where their every wish has been indulged and where there was no discipline. One day, they turn up at work in a foul mood and shout at people.

Which part or parts of the emotional intelligence model are low and creating this problem? If you were their boss, what would be the best thing to do to defuse the problem and help the person improve their performance?

Suggested answer:

From the evidence available, it would seem as if the person concerned has low quality skills in each of the four quadrants of the emotional intelligence model. If you were their boss, it would be good to understand that the development of skills in this case would be likely to be a long journey. The best place to start would probably be in the Self Awareness quadrant, and in the right context and at the right time, encourage the person concerned to become open to receiving feedback from colleagues about the quality of service they provide. Since it would make sense in fact for everyone in the company to routinely give and receive feedback to each other, you might want to consider setting up feedback, possibly on a 360 basis. As their boss, you would be sensitive to the fact that such systems bring with them their own risks, and you might want to consult your staff, including this person, about the best way to do this. There may also be training implications for your staff, including this person.

Scenario 2

Someone in your family displays behaviours associated with a bully. They are driven to achieve great things in their life, and have high expectations of themselves – and others. They believe there is just their way or the highway. This results sometimes in open conflict with others, or in a hostile and fearful atmosphere in the family where people don't say what they really feel.

Which part or parts of the emotional intelligence model are low and creating this problem? As an adult in the family, what's the best thing to do to defuse the problem and help the person improve their performance?

Suggested answer:

This is an example of a *Difficult Conversation* which we explored in chapter ten; and therefore would need all the care we described in this section of the book. It's possible that the person concerned may be under the illusion that they are highly skilled in all four quadrants of the model, but in fact, all the evidence points to them being poorly skilled in all four quadrants. When the time and context are right, it's possible that the best way into a fruitful discussion with them would be about the Self Management quadrant. For example, what would they prefer, rather than spending so much of their life in a bad mood? What gets on their nerves, and how could they develop other options and greater choices, rather than being a victim of bad moods so much?

Scenario 3

One of your relatives is very popular in your family because they're so keen to help everyone else. They're always first to offer help and support to other family members and to neighbours, for example by offering to do their shopping. They're exceptional at anticipating other people's needs. The trouble is that this person gets worn out, and every four – six weeks, feels so exhausted they take time off work, retreat to their bed for a week or so to recuperate. They're exasperated with this pattern, and have asked for your advice.

Which part or parts of the emotional intelligence model are in play here? As a concerned and caring adult in the family, what's the best thing you could do to help this person deal with the underlying issue(s)?

Suggested answer:

This person is probably well skilled in the Social Awareness and the Social Skills quadrants, and may even be reasonably well skilled in the Self Awareness quadrant. Their challenge probably lies in getting more skilled in the Self Management quadrant, ie if they could find more options and choices about how to help others. They probably need to increase their skills and confidence in looking after themselves as well as they look after others. So, at the right time and in the right context, you might want to ask them some questions (in a caring kind of way) about what other options they can think of which result in them not tiring themselves out so much. Maybe they need to include *themselves* on the list of folk they help?

References

Action for Happiness movement,
https://www.actionforhappiness.org
Anderson, I,
www.theguardian.com/world/2020/mar/25/coronavirus-nature-is-sending-us-a-message-says-un-environment-chief
Argyle M and Hills P of Oxford Brookes University, *Oxford Happiness Questionnaire,* in the *Journal of Personality and Individual Differences* 2002
Armstrong T, *The Human Odyssey*, Blackwell's, 2007
Attenborough Sir D, *A Life on the Planet*, Silverback Films and WWF, and the Independent Newspaper, 19 April 2020
Bandler R and Grinder J, *The Structure of Magic Vol 1*, Science and Behavior Books 1975
Bateson G, *Steps to an Ecology of the Mind*, Chandler Publishing, 1972
Benítez-Burraco A, *Psychology Today*, Feb 2017
Berne E, *Games that People Play,* Grove Press, 1964
Briggs K and Myers I, *Gifts Differing,* Consulting Psychologists Press, 1980
Browning G, *Emergenetics,* Collins, 2006
Bull S, *The Game Plan,* Capstone Publishers, 2006
Burmester M and Lindsay J, *Be Kind – a Year of Kindness, One Week at a Time,* 2020

Burns, G. W, 2005, *Naturally happy, naturally healthy: the role of the natural environment in well-being* in Huppert, F. A., Baylis, N., & Keverne, B, 2005, The Science of Well-being, Oxford University Press

Caulfield M, *The Meta Model Demystified,* 2008

Center for Ecoliteracy, *https://www.ecoliteracy.org*

Charvet Shelle R, *Words That Change Minds*, Kendall Hunt, 1995

Covey S, *The 7 Habits of Highly Effective People*, Franklin Covey, 2015

Christie A, *Murder at the Vicarage*, Collins Crime Club, 1930

De Bono E, *Six Thinking Hats,* Little, Brown and Company, 1985

Dement W Dr, *www.end-your-sleep-deprivation.com*

Diener E, *Happiness: Unlocking the Mysteries of Psychological Wealth*, Blackwell Publishing, 2008

Diener E and Robert Biswas-Diener, *Happiness,* Blackwell Publishing, 2008

Drucker P quote: *https://succeedfeed.com/peter-drucker-quotes/*

Ellis A, *How to Live with a Neurotic*, Crown Publishers, 1959

Emmons R, Counting Blessings vs Burdens, Journal of Personality and Social Psychology, 2003

Epictetus, Ancient Greek philosopher (55 – 135 AD)

Ernst F, *Handbook of Listening*, Transactional Analysis Journal, 1971

Faldo N, quote: www.azquotes.com/author/25970-Nick_Faldo

Garcia H, *Ikigai: The Japanese Secret to a Long and Happy Life*, Hutchinson, London 2019

G FEED blog: *http://www.g-feed.com/2020/03/covid-19-reduces-economic-activity.html*

Goleman D et al, *Ecoliterate*, Jossey-Bass, 2012

Griffiths J, *https://edition.cnn.com/2019/05/13/health/carbon-dioxide-world-intl/index.html*

Grinder J, Bandler R et al, *The Structure of Magic Volume 2*, Science and Behavior Books,1989

Harvard University, *https://www.scientificamerican.com/article/what-immunity-to-covid-19-really-means/*

Harvard University, *https://www.health.harvard.edu/staying-healthy/how-to-boost-your-immune-system*

Hatfield E, *Emotional Contagion,* Cambridge University Press, 1994

Helliwell J, Layard R and Sachs J, *World Happiness Report 2019 www.worldhappinessreport/ed/2019*

Holford P and Meek J, *Boost Your Immune System,* Hachette Digital 2010

Holt-Lunstad J, *Social Relationships and Mortality Risk: A Meta-analytic Review* in Plos Medicine, 2010

Johnson M, *www.bestselfology.com*

Korzybski A, *Science and Sanity*, The International Non-Aristotelian Library Publishing company, 4th edition, 1933

Layard R, *Happiness*, Penguin Group, 2005

Layard R, *Can We Be Happier?*, Penguin Random House UK, 2020

LeBourgeois M, in *Pediatrics*, 2017

Lewis B and Pucelik F, *Magic of NLP Demystified*, Metamorphosis Press, 1990

Lyubomirsky S, *The How of Happiness*, Piatkus Press, 2007

McCraty R, *The Impact of New Emotional Self Management, US National Library of Medicine, 1998*

MacLean P, *The Triune Brain in Evolution*, Plenum Press, 1990

Miller G, *The Magical Number 7, Plus or Minus 2*, in Psychological Review 1956

Maslow A, *A Theory of Human Motivation*, 1943

Mauna Loa Observatory, *https://www.esrl.noaa.gov/gmd/obop/mlo*

Mitchell, R, & Popham, F, *Effect of exposure to natural environment on health inequalities,* 2008

Moll J and Zahn R, *Neural Correlates of Trust, Proceedings of the National Academy of Sciences 2007*

Moll J, *The Neural Basis of Human Moral Cognition, in Nature Reviews Neuroscience, 2005*

Moon J, *Learning Journals, Abingdon:Routledge, 2006*

Moore J, *Planting for Butterflies*, 2020

Muir J, *A Thousand Mile Walk to the Gulf*, Boston Houghton Mifflin 1916

Murray J and Jackson A, *Exploring Microcephaly and Human Brain Evolution,* in Developmental Medicine and Child Neurology, May 2012

Maddocks J and Hughes D, *The Impact of Emotional Intelligence in the Workplace*, PSI, 2019

Murray R Sir Prof, in *Psychological Medicine Journal*, 2012

Office for National Statistics (*www.ons.gov.uk*)

Ontario Healthy Communities Commission, *https://www.allianceon.org/Rx-Community-Social-Prescribing-Ontario*

References

Pearson C, *Awaken the Heroes Within,* HarperSanFrancisco, 1991

Peters S, *The Chimp Paradox*, Ebury Publishing, 2012

Pirsig R: *Zen and the Art of Motorcycle Maintenance*, Vintage, 1974

Post S, *Why Good Things Happen to Good People*, Broadway Books, 2007

Rajecki D, *Attitude,* Sunderland MA: Sinauer, 1990

Robbins A, *Awaken the Giant Within,* Penguin Books, 2001

Rock D, *Your Brain at Work*, Harper Collins, 2009

Rolleston J's blog, posted 11 Feb 2013

Santiago Ramon y Cajal, *Degeneration and Regeneration of the Nervous System*, 1887

Seligman M, *Authentic Happiness,* Free Press New York, 2002

Senge P, *The Fifth Discipline*, 1990

Seymour J and O'Connor J, *Introducing NLP*, Mandala, 1990

Shakespeare W, *As You Like It,* Act 2, Scene 7, 1599

Silvia P and O'Brien M, *Self Evaluation and Constructive Functioning, in the Journal of Social and Clinical Psychology,* 2004

Singman S website, *www.human-equation.com*

Smith A, *The Wealth of Nations, 1776*

Twenge Jean M, *The Sad State of Happiness in the United States*, by of San Diego State

US National Institute of Health, *www.imgt.org*

Walker M, *Why We Sleep*, Penguin Books, 2017

Williams M Prof, *www.psych.ox.ac.uk*

Acknowledgments

We are deeply grateful to the following people for their wisdom, teaching, fellowship and encouragement:

John Seymour and all the staff and delegates at JSNLP and JSA from 2002 to 2014
David Sales of First Ascent Group,
www.firstascentgroup.com
Steve Bentley of First Ascent Group,
www.firstascentgroup.com
Neil Almond, 91 Untold, www.91untold.com
John Cooper and Jo Maddocks, Cheltenham
Graham Morris of Training Changes, Cheltenham
Steve Egan
Clay, the artist, at The Art of Clay, Stroud, Glocs, UK
Chris Raisey
Annie Dalton
Margot McCleary
Wyatt Woodsmall
Iain Roberts
Catchwords Writers Group
The staff on the Doctorate in Education course at the University of Gloucestershire from 2008-2014

About the Authors

Pam Keevil

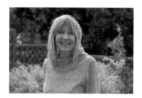

Dr Pam Keevil spent many years as a teacher, headteacher and trainer in both leadership development and personal development. She completed a doctorate at the University of Gloucestershire on the personal development of school leaders in 2014. An MA in Creative and Critical Writing followed in 2016 and her novel *Virgin at Fifty,* a poignant and funny feelgood novel about starting over, was published by Black Pear in 2018. For more information visit www.pamkeevil.com

Peter Keevil

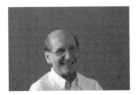

In the last 10 years, Peter Keevil has worked extensively with leaders of lots of organisations in the UK and elsewhere, helping them and their organisations to be the best they can be. Before that, he worked in organisational development in the Higher Education Funding Council for England in Bristol.

He's a qualified coach, NLP master practitioner and a qualified and experienced user of the various tools in the Happiness Toolkit which are described in this book. He has a passion for everything that's explored in this book. He'd be delighted to hear from you and can be contacted at www.linkedin.com/in/peterkeevil/.

We also have a Facebook page where people can, if they wish, share and explore any of the issues raised in this book and the *new and better normal* so many of us now seek. It can be found at: https://www.facebook.com/Finding-Happiness-after-Covid-19-103335108060770

End Notes

[i] http://blog.jeremyrolleston.com/?attachment_id=1167

[ii] https://www.actionforhappiness.org/10-keys-guidebook

[iii] https://commons.wikimedia.org/wiki/File:My_Wife_and_My_Mother-In-Law_(Hill).svg

[iv] https://www.publicdomainpictures.net/se/view-image.php?image=319855&picture=horse-rider-jumping-logo

[v] https://publicdomainvectors.org/en/free-clipart/Vector-image-of-a-brain/8460.html

[vi] https://www.publicdomainpictures.net/cn/view-image.php?image=208416&picture=

[vii] https://www.publicdomainpictures.net/en/view-image.php?image=164684&picture=nonverbal-communication-1

[viii] (https://www.publicdomainpictures.net/en/view-image.php?image=281855&picture=japanese-vintage-art-children

ix
https://www.goodfreephotos.com/%22%3EGood%20Free%2
0Photos%3C/a%3E
x https://www.publicdomainpictures.net/en/view-
image.php?image=292084&picture=angry-woman-silhouette
xi

https://cdn.loc.gov/service/pnp/cph/3a00000/3a04000/3a0400
0/3a04025r.jpg

xii https://www.publicdomainpictures.net/en/view-
image.php?image=4467&picture=spiders-web

Printed in Great Britain
by Amazon